DAVID KATZ, MD, MI   :ector of Yale University's Prevention   .tegrative Medicine Center at Griffin Hospital, and president of the American College of Lifestyle Medicine. Editor in chief of the journal *Childhood Obesity*, he has authored nearly two hundred scientific papers and chapters and fifteen books. Dr. Katz is the recipient of numerous awards and recognitions, including an honorary doctoral degree, and is recognized globally for his expertise in nutrition, weight management, and the prevention of chronic disease. He lives in Connecticut with his family.

STACEY COLINO is the award-winning writer behind *Eat! Move! Play!* and coauthor of *Taking Back the Month*. Her work has appeared in the *Washington Post*, *Newsweek*, *Real Simple*, *Redbook*, *Harper's Bazaar*, and many other publications. She lives with her family in Chevy Chase, Maryland.

Praise for *Disease-Proof*

"David Katz is among my most respected colleagues. When it comes to using lifestyle as medicine, there simply isn't a higher authority. In *Disease-Proof*, Dr. Katz advances a mission we share: empowering people to use what we know about the power of lifestyle to promote health. This is an important book."   —Mehmet Oz, MD

"By offering insight into the hidden and not-so-hidden threats to our collective waistlines and our health and providing step-by-step advice to reverse the current obesity epidemic and the chronic diseases that go with it, *Disease-Proof* will empower readers to take control of their current and future health. Anyone who's interested in protecting themselves and their loved ones from these problems will want to read this book—sooner, not later."   —Dean Ornish, MD, author of *The Spectrum*

"*Disease-Proof* is not only about knowing what to do to stay healthy; it's also about developing the skills to apply that knowledge. Katz and Colino make the skills look easy. I especially appreciate how they encourage readers to take responsibility for the health of others as well as themselves and work toward creating a healthy society for all."
    —Marion Nestle, author of *What to Eat* and professor in the Department of Nutrition, Food Studies, and Public Health at New York University

"Dr. Katz knows how challenging the pursuit of both health and a healthy weight can be. He also has a unique ability to convert his knowledge and insights into practical programs and tools—a talent richly displayed in *Disease-Proof*. If you want to build better health and a better future, this book makes an excellent tool kit."

—David A. Kessler, MD, author of *The End of Overeating*
and former commissioner of the FDA

"*Disease-Proof* is a book we desperately need—a reminder that, in more ways than we may realize, our health is in our hands. Dr. Katz's conclusion that we all have the ability to lead healthier lives is sensible, well-reasoned, empowering, and based on the latest scientific evidence and decades of clinical experience."

—Arianna Huffington, president and editor in chief
of the Huffington Post Media Group

"Comprehensive, accessible, and indispensable, *Disease-Proof* makes a compelling case for how we can reclaim our medical destinies and prevent many of the chronic diseases that are currently afflicting adults and children alike. It's an urgently needed wake-up call for millions of Americans who believe their health is largely beyond their control."

—David Satcher, MD, PhD, former surgeon general
and director of the Centers for Disease Control and Prevention, and
founder of the Satcher Health Leadership Institute,
Morehouse School of Medicine

"The advice in *Disease-Proof*, if applied, will lead to a healthy, vibrant life. Everyone needs this information."

—Christiane Northrup, MD, author of *Women's Bodies,
Women's Wisdom* and *The Wisdom of Menopause*

"*Disease-Proof* uniquely addresses what individuals can do to promote their own health, and what we can and should do together to help us all get there from here. Just about everybody stands to benefit from reading this book."

—Joy Bauer, MS, RD, CDN, nutrition and health expert for the
Today show and author of *Joy Bauer's Food Cures*

DISEASE-PROOF

David L. Katz, MD, MPH,
with Stacey Colino

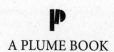

A PLUME BOOK

PLUME
Published by the Penguin Group
Penguin Group (USA) LLC
375 Hudson Street
New York, New York 10014, USA

USA | Canada | UK | Ireland | Australia | New Zealand | India | South Africa | China
penguin.com
A Penguin Random House Company

First published in the United States of America by Hudson Street Press, a member of Penguin
Group (USA) LLC, 2013
First Plume Printing 2014

 REGISTERED TRADEMARK—MARCA REGISTRADA

THE LIBRARY OF CONGRESS HAS CATALOGED THE HUDSON STREET PRESS EDITION AS FOLLOWS:
 Katz, David L., 1963–
 Disease-proof : the remarkable truth about what makes us well / David L. Katz, MD, MPH,
with Stacey Colino.
  pages cm
 Includes bibliographical references and index.
 ISBN 978-1-59463-124-5 (hc.)
 ISBN 978-0-14-218117-1 (pbk.)
 1. Immunity—Nutritional aspects. 2. Health. 3. Self-care, Health. I. Colino, Stacey. II. Title.
 QR185.2.K38 2013
 571.9'6—dc23
                       2013021131

Printed in the United States of America
10 9 8 7 6 5 4 3 2 1

Set in Minion Pro
Original hardcover design by Eve L. Kirch

*To my patients—with gratitude for the rewarding
privilege of sharing skills in pursuit of health.*

Contents

Introduction

When it comes to health, have you ever noticed how the media have a tendency to focus on the latest scary risk factor, a gimmicky new solution, or the bright and shiny promise of a cure (when there never really is one)? That's because diet and health advice in magazines and on TV is, for the most part, designed to get us to read the issue every month or tune in to the program every day. The constantly changing news and advice can leave us feeling downright baffled, but it doesn't bother editors or TV producers in the least. I know this, because I have a bit of insider experience.

In addition to my work as a preventive medicine specialist, I have worked as a columnist for national magazines and as a medical expert for national news shows. One evening several years ago, I was preparing a segment about a new diet study for a TV program the following morning. During a phone call with the writers and producers, we were zipping through the content in a very routine fashion—until I shared what I thought the "punch line" should be. At that point, the senior producer, who had been listening silently, suddenly chimed in, "You can't say that!"

"Why not?" I asked.

"Because you were on the show last week and you said the same thing," she explained. "It will be boring if you repeat the same conclusion."

"Maybe," I replied, "but it happens that fruits and vegetables are *still* good for people!"

This is hardly an uncommon situation; I've encountered it many times in my work. The point here is there's a constant tension in the media between what's new and what's true, what makes for sound science and what makes for provocative headlines or intriguing sound bites. Although I'm sympathetic to the media's challenge to keep their audience engaged, dressing up dull scientific findings to make them sexier, fresher, or more surprising sometimes changes them to the point where the truth can be very hard to recognize.

This phenomenon reminds me of the riveting courtroom scene in the movie *A Few Good Men*, where Tom Cruise's character (a Navy lawyer) is grilling Jack Nicholson's character (a crusty Marine colonel) about whether he ordered a Code Red. At one point Cruise's character hollers that he wants the truth, to which Nicholson's character famously replies, "You can't *handle* the truth!"

The notion that people can't handle the truth if it isn't wrapped in a pretty package is prevalent in the world of health and medicine, too. Can *you* handle it? This is an important question, because if the answer is yes, then you can take control of the master levers of your medical destiny. We can exert incredible power over both the number of years in our lives and the quality of those years. We can help ourselves sidestep illness and health risks and help our children do the same. We can even untwist the implications of our DNA in our favor. The master levers of your personal medical destiny are truly powerful and within your reach.

In the European Prospective Investigation into Cancer and Nutrition (EPIC) Potsdam study, published in 2009, researchers examined four factors—smoking, body weight, physical activity, and diet—among 23,153 German participants, ages thirty-five to sixty-five, and tracked their health effects over the life span. Each healthy lifestyle factor—never smoking, having a body mass index (BMI) lower than 30, performing at least three and a half hours of physical activity per week, and eating a nutritious diet (a high intake of fruits, vegetables, whole-grain bread, and low red meat consumption)—was associated with a decrease in the risk of any chronic disease. Flipping the switch from bad to good on any one of these lifestyle factors was associated with a 50 percent reduced probability of chronic disease. But what was most eye-opening is that participants who had all four healthy factors at the start of the study had a nearly *80 percent* reduced risk of developing any major chronic disease. The reduction in diabetes risk alone was 93 percent. There simply is— and in my opinion, there never will be—no drug to rival that. And to use lifestyle as medicine . . . well, no prescription is required!

It's important to remember that science is all about the slow accumulation of evidence and the gradual evolution of understanding, which sometimes involves confirming time-honored truths. (Yes, fruits and veggies really *are* good for us, just like they were last week and will be next week.) If you put too much stock in the latest media report about what is or isn't good for you or what truly increases or decreases your risk of developing a particular disease, you may end up with a terminal case of health information whiplash. At some point, you may throw up your hands in frustration and tune out the messages entirely, even when they're valid. Clearly, that's not the way it should be.

Contrary to what common assumptions and the media sometimes lead us to believe, our genes do not determine our weight or future health. What they *do* is to tell us about our risks of developing certain diseases. It's about possibility; nothing is set in stone. Our DNA simply cannot forecast that we will get a particular disease, unless it's one that's caused specifically by a genetic mutation (such as Huntington's disease, cystic fibrosis, or sickle cell anemia). We are actually the ones driving the bus on our journeys toward wellness or illness, so don't blame your genes for the future of your health.

Most diseases are not random occurrences but the consequences of the things people do every day. They are the intermediate step between lifestyle habits and infirmity or death. This means that the leading causes of death and disease are largely within our control because they result from what we do or don't do with our feet, our forks, and our fingers— namely, whether we are physically active, consume a healthy diet, or smoke—on a daily basis. With few exceptions, that is the new rule that's been established by groundbreaking research—and it is the central premise of this book. As you've just read, there is now abundant evidence that getting just four things right—not smoking, maintaining a healthy weight, being active, and eating well—could reduce the risk of *all* chronic diseases by 80 percent. That's right: 80 percent! (There are four things on the list, but by eating well and being physically active, you will set yourself up for a healthy weight—so you really need to focus only on three things, with the final one being not smoking.) It's a realization that could, and in my opinion should, remake the way we play the game of life, by inspiring us to make better lifestyle choices. If you do it right, you can write a new story for your future right down to the genetic level. To a preventive medicine specialist like me, this is of profound importance, because apathy and fatalism are among the biggest enemies of health and healing.

Becoming a doctor was a natural choice for me. My father is a doctor, and I knew I wanted to do something that mattered, that felt challenging and rewarding. During my training, I spent a lot of time trying to figure out what kind of doctor I really wanted to be, and I couldn't help but notice that roughly eight out of ten hospitalized patients had serious illnesses, all of which could have been prevented by exercising, eating well, or not smoking. It seemed tragic to me that these people were suffering and shortening their lives—when a more healthful lifestyle could essentially have immunized them against such misery. It was then that the path to my life's work became clear: I started investigating how a doctor becomes an expert in using lifestyle as medicine and how best to leverage nutrition, in particular, to help people avoid getting sick in the first place. The rest, as they say, is history. I have been an internist and a preventive medicine specialist ever since. I rely on both aspects of my training to take care of existing patients—and to try to help as many people as possible avoid becoming my (or any other doctor's) patients in the first place!

Rewrite Your Future

The fact is healthful behaviors create an opportunity to reshuffle the genetic deck in your favor. After all, genes don't affect your health because they're there; they represent a recipe for biological material—including specific proteins that turn those genes on or off—that needs to be made in order to set a disease course into motion. You can change the behavior of your genes, essentially dialing their expression up or down, by modifying your lifestyle. Just because you carry a gene that makes you vulnerable to colon cancer or lung cancer, for example, doesn't mean you'll inevitably develop the disease. If you exercise regularly, stick with a healthy diet, avoid smoking, and maintain a healthy weight, you stand a much better chance of never developing those illnesses, even if other members of your family do.

There are only so many parts to the human body—we can't expect to discover new bones or organs—and the same is true of the skills that will save your life and promote better health and well-being. There is a skill set some people have that enables them, in spite of all the conflicting news and opposing societal forces, to stay lean and maintain good health. They weren't born with this skill; they learned it at some point in their lives, and you can learn it, too. Think of it as an essential tool kit you didn't even know you needed: Once you have it and you master the use of the different tools, you'll have the skills for life.

An 80 percent reduction in the incidence of all chronic disease would certainly count among the most stunning advances in the history of public health. While it's unquestionably a compelling result, it's still just a statistic, and statistics are generally dull, dry, bland—and anonymous. So how can we get passionate about the implications of this idea? Let's consider the personal context of how these risks are playing out in your own world. Have you or any loved ones suffered from a heart attack, a stroke, cancer, or diabetes? Visualize their faces, say their names, and recall what it felt like the day you heard the news that they had developed a life-threatening disease. Remember how upsetting that was?

Now, imagine the faces of friends, colleagues, neighbors, and others as they picture the faces of their loved ones who received similar diagnoses. Think about how they must have been feeling. You probably won't like what you're seeing.

But wait: Now imagine if eight out of ten of us who are reflecting on that personal anguish never got that dreadful news because it never happened. Mom did not get cancer. Your close friend or colleague did not have a heart attack. Grandpa did not have a stroke. You didn't develop diabetes. That's a far more upbeat and inspiring picture, isn't it? Even more inspiring: It's possible, if we all do our part individually, to reclaim control of our feet, forks, and fingers. The key is to transform what's now known about the potential to combat chronic disease into action, because knowledge isn't power unless it's put to good use.

Your Body's Second Chance

When I ask my patients why they've come to see me, the answer is always to get better if something is wrong, or to get advice about staying healthy if nothing's currently bothering them. My second question is "Why do you care about being healthy? What is health for?"

Usually these questions are met with silence. No one really thinks about the fact that health is *for* something, but it is. It's for living the life you want and deserve, for feeling good and functioning at your best. It's not a trial, a penance, or a punishment. It's a reward and a return on your investment in yourself (a return that more than justifies the investment, by the way). That's true of the money we put aside to secure our futures or pay for our kids' educations, and it's certainly true of the effort devoted to improving our health. After all, your life will be better if you have good health. And if you pay it forward by sharing your health-promoting, disease-fighting strategies with loved ones, your life will be better still because the people you love will share good health with you.

It requires effort and practice to make these skills automatic, especially given the world we live in. We didn't choose to be born into an environment that promotes obesity, but here we are, nevertheless. We did not choose to find ourselves in a world awash in highly palatable, energy-dense, convenient foods. And while we did not choose to be among the first generation of *Homo sapiens* that could count on technology to do everything for us, in areas ranging from work to recreational pursuits, once again, here we are. You don't need to be gluttonous to overeat or lazy to underexercise and gain weight in the modern world; you simply need to live in the modern world, which is why obesity and chronic disease are not exceptions—they are now the norm.

There's a place for both personal responsibility and public policy in fixing what ails our collective health. While you're waiting for the world to change, it is possible to steer the course of your own and your family's health in a better direction, and this book will show you how. Part call to action, part blueprint for healthy living, this book examines the specific factors that are contributing to the epidemics of obesity and chronic diseases in our culture and, most important, provides the tools that will empower you to make health-promoting changes so that you can better manage your weight, bolster your natural immunity, nip life-altering illnesses before they even have a chance to bud, and possibly even undo previous damage from existing disease. For the first time ever, you will gain an entire tool kit that will enable you to seize control over your medical destiny for good. It's like riding a bicycle: once you know how, you never forget.

In the chapters that follow, you will learn how to fortify your willpower and build the skills that will help you improve your eating habits at home and on the road, your food-shopping and cooking habits, and your level of physical activity. You'll learn how to retrain your taste buds to prefer healthier foods, discover physical activities you enjoy and fit them into your life, and embrace the gift of physical vitality. And you'll find out how to improve other aspects of your lifestyle—including your sleep, stress, pain, and social connections—so they can enhance your eating and exercise habits. Best of all, you'll be able to tailor a plan that's specific to your situation and needs. Let's get started!

DISEASE-PROOF

• One •

The Power to Nurture Nature

In our culture, we tend to refer to hospitals, clinics, physicians, nurses, and other clinicians collectively as a "health care system." This may cause you to think that someone or something else—perhaps a doctor, or a drug or other treatment—has the ultimate control over your health. But that's just not the case. By and large, the system in place is a "disease care system," not a health care system. Disease care is important when you are sick and in need of treatment. But only rarely are professional clinical services actually related to the promotion of health. That power resides almost entirely with you.

A recent report from the Centers for Disease Control and Prevention (CDC) suggested that we owe our increasing life spans largely to cutting-edge biomedical advances, rather than to our own personal choices. The National Center for Health Statistics at the CDC reported that overall life expectancy in the United States has increased to the unprecedented high of 77.9 years overall, with women, as ever, outliving men with an average life expectancy of 80.4, compared to 75.3 years for men.

In 2012, *The Lancet* published a comprehensive report stating that life expectancy is increasing in most places around the globe, due to various advances in modern medicine and public health. The bad news: There is an increasing burden of chronic disease beginning at ever-younger ages in most developed and developing countries. The result is more years of illness, something that's especially prominent here in the United States.

One article in the report addresses a standard of measurement called "HALE"—which means "healthy life expectancy." In the United States in 2010, healthy life expectancy for men was 65.0 years (roughly 11 years less than actual life expectancy), and for women it was 67.4 years (roughly 13 years less than actual life expectancy). What is most disturbing about these numbers is the gap between actual and healthy life expectancy, a significant span of years spent living with the serious burdens of chronic disease and disability. This is a very dubious trade-off.

Both the *Lancet* study and the CDC are sources of authoritative data indicating that rates of obesity, diabetes, and chronic disease are at an all-time high in the United States (and, increasingly, the world). The math here is not very complicated. If life expectancy and chronic disease rates are rising in tandem, it means we are living longer, but in a sicker state. In the United States, more than 75 percent of Medicare expenditures—an annual total of many hundreds of billions of dollars— is for the care of chronic diseases. But it doesn't have to be this way. Only *we* can build actual health at its origins. Each of us already holds the potential power to change the course of our health across our life span— but we need the right skills to put that power to use.

Yet many people continue to revisit the question of how much of our collective and personal health risks are due to nature (genetics) versus nurture (environment). This issue received renewed attention in the last decade as we entered the genomic age. With the mysteries of the human genome unraveled, it seemed likely we would soon be "fixing" the causes of diseases with genetic engineering. That simply hasn't happened. But a funny thing has happened on the way: Increasingly, research has revealed the extent to which environment, and our lifestyle habits in particular, can affect our risk of developing chronic, life-threatening diseases, even at their genetic origins. In other words, we've been looking down the wrong path and asking the wrong questions. The reality is, we actually don't need new scientific breakthroughs or Nobel Prizes to fix genetic causes of major diseases. We already have that power, and it's time for us to reclaim it, individually and as a society.

After all, the national obesity epidemic is bringing serious health consequences to us personally and to our loved ones, and creating skyrocketing costs in health care expenses and lost productivity to the nation (including high rates of absenteeism, inefficient work, and failure to advance in the workplace). Meanwhile, approximately 17 percent of the medical costs in the United States can be blamed on obesity, according to recent research that suggests the nation's (over)weight problem may be having nearly twice the impact on medical spending as previously believed. Excess weight is not the only problem; so are the chronic diseases—some life-threatening (such as heart disease and diabetes), others life-compromising (such as osteoarthritis and chronic heartburn)—that tend to come with it. According to the CDC, approximately 35 percent of adults in the United States are currently obese (defined as having a body mass index, or BMI, of 30 or higher), and a new report suggests that this figure will climb to 42 percent by 2030, which would cost the United States an additional $549.5 billion in medical expenses over the next two decades. That's more than the annual U.S. military budget and more than fifteen years of funding for the National Institutes of Health! In other words, we stand to squander the equivalent of more than a decade and a half of funding for the world's premier biomedical research laboratory on the totally preventable costs of getting fatter.

If current trends persist, the CDC is projecting that one in three adults (roughly one hundred million people) will have diabetes by the year 2050. Meanwhile, hospitalization rates for ischemic stroke (the most common kind, caused by a decrease in blood supply to the brain) are already rising among five- to fourteen-year-olds, according to a recent CDC study, largely because of the prevalence of childhood obesity and the hypertension that often comes with it. Stroke and ischemic heart disease are not expected in such a young age group, but they are occurring with increasing and alarming frequency. Furthermore, the latest research suggests that the precursors for adult heart disease—including atherosclerosis, hypertension, diabetes, cholesterol abnormalities, and metabolic syndrome—actually begin in childhood, and that childhood obesity plays a considerable role.

The unfortunate truth is that childhood obesity rates have been rising at a disturbing speed for decades, and although recent data suggest a possible plateau, obesity is seen in younger and younger children, and is increasingly severe. Officially, approximately 17 percent of children in the United States are considered obese (their BMI is at or above the 95th percentile for their age and gender), and an additional 10 to 15 percent are considered overweight (their BMI is at or above the 85th percentile for their age and gender). In some minority groups, this figure rises to 50 percent. Even these alarming statistics, however, may fail to reflect the true rate of obesity in children, because the very definitions of obesity and overweight in childhood have been devised to be more exclusive than inclusive, in part to minimize the number of children who are encumbered by this stigmatizing label. Casual observations of the world around us would suggest that the actual rate of overweight children is considerably higher.

Less than a generation ago, type 2 diabetes was routinely referred to as "adult-onset diabetes." In the past two decades, type 2 diabetes has been transformed from a condition occurring almost exclusively at or after middle age into a childhood epidemic affecting children as young as six, largely because of lifestyle factors. Besides the inherent health risks (including increased risk of heart attack, blindness, amputation, and kidney disease), children who have the condition are at greater risk for heart disease and other chronic diseases. Because children with type 2 diabetes will have it for more years during their lives than adults who develop it, there's more time for them to suffer from complications. As the American Academy of Pediatrics (AAP) noted recently, this may be the first generation of children destined to have a shorter life expectancy than their parents. That's a sobering reality, indeed.

The scenario just described is a clear and omnipresent danger—and it's knocking at your door, stalking you and your children. That's why it's time to take it personally. For the past two decades, every analysis of the available research has reaffirmed the finding that feet, forks, and fingers are the indisputable master levers of medical destiny. While this research has also suggested that as the toll of tobacco use has been declining in recent years—persistence of the habit has stalled, with approximately 20 percent of the population continuing to smoke—the toll of eating badly and forgoing exercise has been rising, in some cases dramatically.

We have two options: Either we prevent these forecasted trends from happening, or we succumb to them. It's really that simple. A third option for those who already have these diseases is to reverse them or better manage them with healthy lifestyle habits, which will improve long-term health. But knowledge is power only if you know what to do with it. Right now, there's a good chance you don't know how much power you have or how to use it. (This book will change that!) This has certainly been true of most of my patients over the years.

Several years ago, a young man named Doug came to see me to find out if he was at risk of having a heart attack, and if so, what he could do about it. His motivation was both common and powerful: fear. His father, age fifty, had just had a heart attack—fortunately, not fatal—so Doug, who was twenty-seven, had started thinking seriously about his own health for the first time. He thought that the power to avoid what had happened to his dad resided with me, a fairly common assumption—but he was wrong. The power to prevent a heart attack was his alone.

When I asked about his lifestyle, I learned that Doug didn't smoke, nor did his father. But prior to the heart attack, his father had been sedentary, had eaten rather poorly, and was substantially overweight. Doug was overweight and fairly sedentary, too. He also ate as poorly as his father did—a diet heavy on fast food and processed foods, light on foods that come directly from nature.

This young man came to me afraid of dying and expected me to fix things. He thought I might check his blood pressure and cholesterol and perhaps order a cardiogram and a stress test. When I asked what he thought we might do if his blood pressure was elevated and whether he'd want me to prescribe a drug right away, he said he didn't want to take medication if he didn't have to.

So we began discussing other options. He knew that exercise, weight loss, and less sodium in his diet were important measures for controlling blood pressure. He also knew that eating oats, vegetables, fruit, and fish would be good for his cholesterol levels; that fried foods were bad for it; and that exercise and weight loss would help, too.

I ran some tests, and it turned out his blood pressure was normal but on the high side, and his blood lipid levels were also normal, if not quite ideal. Doug realized his father had probably been in a similar position at twenty-seven, but that all of these health risks tend to increase as a person gets older. He also realized that actually implementing the behaviors he knew would improve his blood pressure and cholesterol would help keep these measures in the normal range.

To me, the obvious question was: What was Doug waiting for? Since he knew about many of the lifestyle factors that could do the same job as medicine, why wasn't he putting them to use? Maybe he needed me to confirm that he was right about what he should do. Maybe he needed some help figuring out how to take action. Maybe he needed me for motivation. In part, I think he came to see me because he had bought into the prevailing perspective that our high-tech, there's-a-pill-or-procedure-for-everything culture propagates: The power over health resides mostly with doctors and the health care system. But the power to avoid his father's fate did not reside mostly with me. It resided overwhelmingly with him.

I'm pleased to report that after a series of appointments, Doug took that simple revelation and put it to good use. The last time I saw him, he was leaner, fitter, healthier, and far less concerned about his future—because he had taken his medical destiny into his own hands, where it belonged.

A Convenient (and Important!) Medical Truth

For many years, the nature/nurture debate has invited us to wonder if what mattered more was the hand we were dealt or how we played that hand. The startling truth is: You get to reshuffle the deck! The power of your lifestyle can reshape your destiny at the very level of your genes. Healthy eating and exercise habits can reduce your risk of developing a chronic disease, and sometimes it can reverse a disease you already have or prevent a recurrence.

In 1993 a paper entitled "Actual Causes of Death in the United States," by Drs. J. Michael McGinnis and William Foege was published in the prestigious *Journal of the American Medical Association*, or *JAMA*. There, McGinnis and Foege described the obvious revelation that we, in the medical profession, had all overlooked: that the diseases we had long listed as the leading causes of death—heart disease, cancer, stroke, pulmonary illness, and diabetes—are not truly *causes*. These diseases are *the results* or *effects* of how people live. When someone dies of, say, a heart attack, it is not very illuminating to blame the cause of death on disease of the cardiovascular system, is it? What we all really want to know is what caused the cardiovascular disease.

The answer was readily available, but someone had to go looking for it, and that's what Drs. McGinnis and Foege did. They found that, overwhelmingly, premature death and chronic disease were attributable to just ten behaviors: tobacco use, dietary pattern, physical activity level, alcohol consumption, exposure to germs, exposure to toxins, use of firearms, sexual behavior, motor vehicle crashes, and use of illicit drugs. The list of ten was dominated by the top three: tobacco use, dietary pattern, and physical activity level, which accounted for nearly eight hundred thousand premature deaths in 1990—about 80 percent of the total! When scientists from the CDC reassessed this landscape a decade later, they found that relatively little had changed. Across the span of a decade, injudicious use of feet, forks, and fingers remained the primary causes of poor health.

More recently, researchers from the CDC examined the links between three healthy lifestyle behaviors—consuming a healthy diet, getting adequate physical activity, and not smoking—and the risk of premature death among 8,375 adults in the United States. Over a period of five-plus years, the physically active folks had a 51 percent lower risk of dying, those who simply consumed a healthy diet had a 23 percent lower risk, and nonsmokers had a 56 percent lower chance of dying. Those who followed all three healthy behaviors had an 82 percent reduction in premature death from any disease. Meanwhile, a group of researchers from Norway and the United Kingdom found much the same thing in a study of more than 5,000 adults in the United Kingdom, reported in the *Archives of Internal Medicine* in April 2010.

As it turns out, we are all making life-or-death decisions every single day in terms of what we choose to put into our bodies and how we choose to use them. Those decisions truly do reverberate all the way to our DNA. In 2008 there was an illuminating trial called the Gene Expression Modulation by Intervention with Nutrition and Lifestyle (GEMINAL) study, which was developed by my friend Dr. Dean Ornish and his colleagues at the University of California, San Francisco. It involved thirty men with early-stage prostate cancer who were eligible to be observed carefully for disease progression without undergoing surgery, radiation, or chemotherapy. A bit of background: Some prostate cancers progress and metastasize throughout the body; when this occurs, the disease is devastating and often lethal. But some tumors of the prostate are indolent; in essence, they just sit there, doing nothing. As many as 80 percent of men in the United States who die after age eighty have prostate cancer, but they die with it rather than from it.

The GEMINAL study took advantage of this indolent variety of prostate cancer to assess the effects of a lifestyle intervention, without the confounding influences of medical or surgical cancer treatments. The lifestyle changes included a low-fat, plant-based, whole foods diet; stress management techniques; moderate exercise; and participation in a psychosocial support group. The study lasted three months, and many of the usual measures of overall health were tracked: weight, blood pressure, cholesterol levels, and so on. They all improved significantly, as one would expect. Levels of PSA (prostate-specific antigen), a tumor marker for prostate cancer, improved, but only trivially.

What made this study groundbreaking is that it measured health markers beyond the list of usual suspects. Using advanced laboratory techniques, the investigators measured the effects of the intervention at the level of the genes—and what they found was remarkable. By examining prostate biopsy specimens before and after the three-month intervention, they saw significant changes in gene activity. Roughly fifty genes associated with cancer suppression became more active in generating RNA (a nucleic acid that essentially acts as a messenger carrying instructions from DNA), and nearly five hundred genes associated with cancer progression became less active. The pattern of change observed in gene activity was consistently and decisively associated with lower risk of cancer development and progression. In other words, diet and lifestyle exerted a powerful effect within the double helix of DNA itself!

Since this study showed a change in the behavior of genes in people who already had cancer—a change in genes that would be expected to slow or prevent cancer growth—this study suggests that lifestyle measures have the power actually to reverse cancer. If a cancer is essentially "stopped in its tracks" by a change in gene behavior—and if that cancer never grows, spreads, or causes discernible harm—it's really just as good as a cure. Of course, we will need longer-term studies to prove that this effect is possible, but the research is already suggesting it.

While this study is unique, it's becoming less so all the time. Other investigators have produced similar results, showing changes in gene expression with lifestyle interventions. Such studies, which are proliferating quickly, suggest potential benefits across a wide array of conditions—including breast, colon, and other cancers; heart disease; stroke; diabetes; and more. We've long known that if you're overweight, losing weight tends to be good for your health, and if you are overweight *and* have insulin resistance, weight loss can improve insulin sensitivity and protect against diabetes. In fact, the Diabetes Prevention Program, a multicenter clinical research study, was designed to investigate whether lifestyle measures or treatment with the oral diabetes drug metformin could prevent type 2 diabetes in high-risk individuals. It found that following a balanced, sensible diet and getting moderate physical activity led to an average loss of 7 percent of body weight, which in turn reduced the risk of subsequent diabetes by a full 58 percent. By contrast, those taking only the drug reduced their risk by only 31 percent. That's right: A modest upgrade of lifestyle and moderate weight loss prevented nearly two out of three people who were at high risk from getting diabetes, nearly double the results of simply taking a drug.

This is impressive, to be sure, but the latest genetic research tops it. More recently, a study called GENOBIN (Gene Expression in Obesity and Insulin Resistance) has shown that long-term weight loss also changes the genes that are involved in cell death. Down-regulating the activity of such genes essentially applies an anti-disease, antiaging salve directly to your DNA. It's like putting on a protective coat of armor from the inside out.

Indeed, if you change your lifestyle, particularly your eating and exercise habits, you can change the expression of your genes even after you've been diagnosed with a disease, and/or modify your risk of experiencing a recurrence. While I don't measure gene expression in my practice—nobody does in a clinical setting—I have seen many patients take matters into their own hands after a grim diagnosis and improve their health greatly by adopting a healthy lifestyle. A former patient named Dale comes to mind. When Dale was in his mid-fifties, he worked too hard, slept too little, dealt poorly with stress, got little to no exercise, and, most important, consumed an unhealthy diet (lots of fried foods and red meat, and too few vegetables, whole grains, and fruit). After suffering a heart attack that landed him in the ER, then the critical care unit, Dale had to have his occluded arteries opened up with a cardiac catheterization. His cardiologist prescribed lots of medication and followed him closely, and then Dale decided to adopt a healthy lifestyle.

By the time we met, Dale was in his early sixties and had already revamped his diet and become physically active. At our last visit for routine care, he was seventy-three and looked like Jack LaLanne at the peak of his vitality—fit, strong, and chiseled. His blood pressure and cholesterol levels were perfect. The results of his stress test were optimal, and he was the very picture of health. The only medication he was taking was aspirin. He just didn't need anything else.

I have seen similar reversals of fortune with patients who've been diagnosed with diabetes or cancer and changed their lifestyle habits—a pattern that's supported by research. In a recent review of the medical literature on the link between physical activity and disease outcomes among cancer survivors, researchers at Bellarmine University in Louisville, Kentucky, found that regular exercise is associated with a decreased risk of breast cancer recurrence. Moreover, an analysis of observational studies by researchers from the National Cancer Survivorship Initiative in the United Kingdom suggests that a low-fat, high-fiber diet may protect against recurrence of breast, colorectal, and prostate cancer. The evidence is even stronger for physical activity with a dose-response relationship, meaning the more that cancer survivors exercise, the lower their risk of a recurrence.

Putting Your Fingers to Better Use

When it comes to smoking, there's also an opportunity to undo previous damage—if you kick the habit. While smoking isn't as prevalent these days, about 20 percent of adults in the United States still do smoke, and here's something you should know: Smoking cigarettes damages just about every organ in the body and accounts for at least 30 percent of all deaths from cancer, according to the American Cancer Society. It also increases the risks of heart disease, stroke, aneurisms, osteoporosis, macular degeneration (an eye disease that causes blindness), and other chronic diseases. So if you smoke, quit. Really, it's nonnegotiable.

Fortunately, there is a variety of aids that can make it a bit easier to kick the habit. These include group support programs, nicotine replacement therapy (gums, patches, nasal sprays, inhalers, and lozenges), medications (such as certain antidepressants), hypnosis, and acupuncture.

Your best bet is to talk to your doctor about which one(s) might be suitable for you—then look at the calendar and set a quit date!

The sooner you quit, the better it will be for your health, but it's never too late. It also may take a few attempts before your effort sticks. In a recent study involving 113,752 women and 88,496 men between the ages of twenty-five and seventy-nine, researchers at the Center for Global Health Research, in Toronto, found that the risk of dying from any cause was three times higher among current smokers than among those who'd never smoked, and life expectancy was about a decade shorter among current smokers. Here's the real surprise: The research found that quitting smoking restores life expectancy more than you might think. Smokers who quit between the ages of twenty-five and thirty-four regained all ten years they would have lost if they'd continued smoking; those who quit between thirty-five and forty-four gained back nine of those lost years, and those who kicked the habit between forty-five and fifty-four gained back six years of lost life expectancy. So quitting at any age really can help you stave off premature death.

Harnessing the Power of Epigenetics

Each of us was born with particular genes; it's a fact of life. But our modern understanding of genetics and genomics has evolved to emphasize the role of "epigenetics"—how genes are influenced by *their* environment. Quite simply, their environment is . . . *you*! As we've already seen, the way you live—in terms of your eating, exercise, sleep, stress management, and other habits—changes the environment of your genes, and that in turn changes what they do. Specific genes may make you more prone to inflammation (which can damage tissue throughout your body), aging (a gradual deterioration of function at the cellular and organ levels), degeneration (wear and tear to the lining of your arteries, or to your cartilage or joints), and oxidation (a process akin to "rusting" in the body). The expression of these genes is, in turn, influenced by the environment inside your body. Genes that may cause you to make more or less insulin, cholesterol, or white blood cells are also all influenced by your lifestyle.

If you develop wholesome habits, you can give the DNA you were born with a second chance—a do-over, so to speak—to move in a healthier direction. You can reshuffle the genetic deck in your favor with healthful behaviors—enough to reduce the likelihood of a bad health outcome by 80 percent. Those are shockingly good odds! No medicine, supplement, or medical intervention can even come close to delivering results like that. *Not even close.*

In the short term, using your fork to feed yourself more wholesome foods and your feet to put your body into motion (and keep it there) can lead to more immediate benefits, including better mood and mental clarity, improved sleep, more energy, less pain and stress, and a greater overall sense of well-being. In a recent review of the medical literature, researchers at the University of Auckland, in New Zealand, found that light- to moderate-intensity exercise even reduces cigarette cravings and withdrawal symptoms in people who are trying to kick the habit. How can you argue with this many feel-good perks?

Even if you already have a chronic illness, your prognosis will almost certainly be better if you take good care of yourself. It's true of cancer, and it's true of hypertension and diabetes, too. For some people, even optimal use of their feet and forks may not be quite enough to avoid hypertension or cholesterol abnormalities, for example; they may also require medication to treat their condition, but healthy lifestyle habits will allow the medication to work more effectively.

The most important question for you to ponder now is: How effectively am I using the levers that control my medical future? If you're like most people, the answer is: not well. The answer may even be: not at all. That's not your fault. It's really the norm in our culture and our society. But it doesn't have to stay that way for you and your family. It's time to establish a new normal! The journey to get there begins with willpower. You need to care. If you *don't* care about creating better health, a better life, a better future for your children; more years in your life and more vibrancy in your years; or an 80 percent reduction in the likelihood of *ever* getting *any* serious chronic disease—you should probably close this book now.

Caring is not enough, though. People talk a lot about *will*power; they don't talk nearly enough about *skill*power. You might *want* to pilot a 747, but it's best not to try it if you don't have the expertise. You might *want* to see the world from the top of Mount Everest, but you can't even consider making the ascent without developing serious mountaineering skills. Getting to wellness is a lot less difficult, but it, too, requires skill-power, which will be explored in detail in the next chapter.

The real epiphany about losing weight, upgrading your lifestyle, and finding good health is not one isolated ingredient someone can patent and sell to you. It's the big picture. The active ingredient in a healthy diet is not vitamin E or resveratrol; it's real, healthy food. The most effective tool in health-promoting exercise is not some fancy gadget but moving your body regularly. You can put together the ultimate tool kit for avoiding illness and embracing good health. Amassing the proper tools and mastering the ability to use them adeptly will give you what you need to reach the prize of better health, greater longevity, and more vitality—*that* is the real-world revelation.

Two

Where There's a Will . . . There's a Way to Build Skillpower

Former presidential candidate Mike Huckabee is a friend of mine, and while we differ quite a bit in our perspectives on politics and policy, we respect each other. (For the record, we both think it would be nice if that happened more often in our society.) Mike and I met when he was governor of Arkansas and chairman of the National Governors Association. He had taken up the cause of addressing childhood obesity, and I was privileged to be among those he called upon to help advance the mission, which brought the fringe benefit of getting to know him personally. One day, as we jogged together through the heart of Little Rock and past the Clinton Library, I commented that I felt a unique sense of security jogging on streets with the governor who was in charge of them. As we were crossing a busy intersection, he remarked, "Well, remember that about half of these people voted for the other guy!"

At the time, Mike had recently lost more than 100 pounds, an impressive feat that took him from dangerously obese to running marathons, which he chronicled in his inspiring book *Quit Digging Your Grave with a Knife and Fork*. Mike attributed his success to taking personal responsibility for his weight issues, and there's no doubt he did so, and he deserves plenty of credit for that. But as I pointed out in some of our discussions, he had more than the average person's resources, including a personal chef and a staff at his disposal. As governor, all he had to do was make a call, and any health care professional in the state (if not the country) would trip over himself trying to offer help. In fact, Mike enjoyed the expert guidance of, among others, Dr. Joe Thompson, an obesity expert and surgeon general for the state of Arkansas.

I pointed out to the governor—and continue to point out to others every chance I get—that the playing field of opportunity for taking personal responsibility for body weight and health is not a level one. Compare the governor's situation, for instance, with that of a single mom who works fourteen hours a day and has little help with her kids. Maybe she needs to lose weight and become more active to thwart diseases she may be at risk for. But her work hours make it impossible for her to spend time outdoors in daylight, and after work, she's eager to get home to be with her kids. Sure, we could tell this woman she needs to lift herself up by her bootstraps, but the painful reality is she doesn't have the right boots! And she may not be able to afford them, either.

In our culture, we like to say that "where there's a will, there's a way." It's certainly a nice thought, but in fact it's not possible to achieve every goal you set your sights on, if you don't have the wherewithal or the opportunity to strive for them. The truth is, where there's a will, there's really just a will. It's an important first step, but it's not enough. You also need a way, one that you can identify and consistently be able to follow.

In the chapters that follow, you'll learn how to develop the requisite skillpower that will help you conquer lifestyle challenges presented by the modern world. Of course, it would be ideal if the road to wellness contained fewer potholes, bumps, and detours—if it were a path of lesser resistance so the burden of the journey didn't fall entirely on your shoulders. But we can't just wait for the world to change, not with our health on the line every day. We need to change our own behavior in the meantime, and deal with the world as it is now.

The first step, then, is to address the issue of willpower, the inner strength that allows you to control and carry out your decisions, wishes, and plans. Willpower also encompasses your ability to use your desire for a goal as a force to initiate change and move in the direction of the prize. You can thank your brain's prefrontal cortex for these functions: Once relegated to controlling physical movements, it has evolved to take up a larger portion of the brain. Now it also controls your attention, your thoughts, and your feelings, which makes it even better at controlling your actions. Without the prefrontal cortex, none of us would have an ounce of self-control. Yet, despite being highly evolved human beings, a 2012 survey by the American Psychological Association tells us that adults in the United States consistently report that a lack of willpower is the primary reason they don't meet their goals to lose weight, save money, exercise more, or make other lifestyle changes.

The *Spider-Man* comics and movies gave us the notion that with great power comes great responsibility. Peter Parker's uncle Ben gives him this sage counsel; it's a noble maxim and one we should embrace in the health arena, among other areas of our lives. But there is, or should be, a corollary to that adage, and it goes like this: You have to be empowered before you can take responsibility. Otherwise, you may have the will but lack the way. That's a formula for serious frustration and a set-up for failure.

The Pressure System Model

I have studied the underpinnings of behavior change for nearly twenty years in my lab at the Yale-Griffin Prevention Research Center. Many years back, my colleagues and I developed a behavior modification concept called the Pressure System Model, and we have since gone on to publish results of studies based on it. The term *pressure system* comes, of course, from meteorology, where it is used to tell us what weather to expect. Like the wind, our behavior also blows from high to low, with two pressure systems involved: motivation and resistance.

If motivation for changing your behavior is high, and there is no resistance (in other words, it's easy to do), you will almost certainly achieve your goal. On the other hand, if motivation is absent or low, there's no wind beneath your wings or anywhere else. In this case it doesn't matter whether resistance is high or low, because without motivation to alter your behavior, you simply won't bother to try. If you aren't interested in working out, it doesn't matter if you have loads of free time, full-time child care, support from friends and family, or even a home gym; you're still unlikely to get moving.

In between these polar-opposite scenarios is the situation many people are in right now. You may want the prize—whether it's losing weight, getting fit, increasing your vitality, living longer, or undoing damage from diabetes, hypertension, or another condition you already have—but it's just too hard. If motivation is fairly high (or even quite high) but resistance is even higher, you won't change your behavior—not because you lack the will, but because you lack the way to attain your goals. The purpose of the Pressure System Model is to help determine whether what stands between you and better health is a lack of motivation, a series of obstacles, or both. There's no need to fix what isn't broken, but you do need to focus your attention and efforts on fixing what *is* broken, so you can improve your chances of reaching your goals. The value of this model lies in its simplicity: You need only to consider why you want to change your habits and what stands in your way of doing so. By evaluating whether you need to raise your motivation, overcome substantial resistance, or both, you can identify which strategies will best support your efforts to improve the way you use your feet and forks.

Let's return to the example of Mike Huckabee. During his 2008 presidential campaign, I couldn't help but notice that he had gained back a considerable portion of the weight he had lost. I very much doubt that his will for controlling his weight and improving his health had gone away. What did go away were all the resources that had helped him get there in the first place. In other words, "the way" got much, much harder because he faced more resistance. So the will that had been enough under one set of circumstances was not enough under a different set.

Life is like that for everyone. Simply put, you need to have enough will to overcome the impediments that reside along the way to whatever result or goal you are seeking. How much will is enough depends on the size and quantity of those obstacles or impediments. If there are many impediments and/or they're very large, you will need either to care so passionately and fervently about your mission that nothing will stop you from reaching your destination, or to find ways to overcome or get around and past those obstacles. Most of us reside in the latter camp.

To do that, you will need skillpower—the skills, strategies, resources, and tools that will empower you to overcome the obstacles you face. As it happens, having ample skillpower reduces the amount of willpower required to get to the prize. One without the other is ineffective; together, they provide a powerful one-two punch for getting the job done.

A case in point: In a study designed to prevent type 2 diabetes through lifestyle modifications, researchers at Aston University in the United Kingdom examined the effects of a motivational intervention (designed to increase self-efficacy: the conviction that you can get the job done), a volitional intervention (focused on action planning and coping strategies), or a combination of the two. While the motivational arm did increase the participants' motivated thoughts, it was the combination intervention that helped the participants significantly decrease their fat intake and increase their frequency of exercise and the amount of fruit and vegetables they consumed. In a similar study, researchers at Coventry University in the United Kingdom tested whether a motivational intervention, a volitional intervention, or a combined approach was more effective in helping people embark on and stick to a regular walking program. Once again, the combined approach won out. Besides leading to a significant increase in walking behavior among participants in that group, it also increased self-efficacy substantially, which would likely help them maintain their gains in physical activity.

One of the great demonstrations of the strength, and limits, of willpower is the time-honored tradition of the New Year's resolution. To the extent that human beings continue to make resolutions, this is an example of the triumph of hope over experience. On one level, I rather like what that says about our collective sense of optimism! The practice of making New Year's resolutions has been around a long time. The ancient Babylonians practiced the resolution craft and, according to historians, often made a New Year's pledge to return borrowed farm equipment. The

Romans, who named January after their forward- and backward-facing god, Janus, often took stock of their past behaviors and vowed to make improvements in the year ahead.

However the Babylonians and ancient Romans fared in their times, we in the modern age tend to do rather poorly in making our resolutions stick. Most research suggests that fewer than half of New Year's resolutions—which often focus on eating healthier food, losing weight, exercising more, and quitting smoking—survive past February, and at least one study suggests that less than 20 percent last two years or longer. To be honest, I'm surprised the numbers are that good. On the one hand, this shows that willpower is, indeed, powerful. At the very least, it gets legions of people to commit every year to trying something they know is important, even though it's hard work.

And let's face it: It takes real effort to eat well and be active, especially in the modern world. It's incredibly challenging to take personal responsibility for eating right or exercising when your environment doesn't support such actions. Throughout most of human history, calories were relatively scarce and difficult to get, and physical activity was unavoidable. No one needed willpower to avoid eating too much and moving too little in a world like that; eating the right amount and being active were called survival. But we have created a modern world in which it's easy to be sedentary and to consume excess calories.

Like all creatures, human beings have innate defenses against certain environmental hazards as well as against starvation. We also have a high tolerance for physical exertion. In other words, we are built to adapt well to situations that involve consuming few calories and doing lots of exercise. But we have no way to defend ourselves against the effects of caloric excess and the lure of the couch—it's simply not in our genetic makeup. When eating too much and moving too little are not only possible but easy, they tend to happen, which is how we've landed together in the world of epidemic obesity and the chronic diseases that tend to go with it.

It's a tall order to expect willpower to overcome all this, which is why skillpower matters so much (and why so much of this book is about *that*). But the first critical skill is having the will, caring in a way that is truly constructive. Will equals wanting. Willpower is using that desire to initiate action. In other words, willpower is the use of will as a force for change. So truly getting power from will is a notch up from simply having the will. In their book, *Willpower*, psychologist Roy Baumeister and John Tierney point out that each of us has a single well of willpower to draw from—there isn't a separate one for your eating habits, another for exercise, one for work, and another for your personal relationships—and the well gradually becomes depleted as you use it. As Baumeister notes, "willpower, like a muscle, becomes fatigued from overuse," but it "can also be strengthened over the long term through exercise."

Indeed, the human brain is a highly malleable organ, and with practice, it can be trained to get better at performing crossword puzzles, playing the piano, learning new computer programs, and even exercising self-control. To change our lifestyle, the first steps are to train our willpower muscle and make more conscious choices while also developing skillpower that we can put to good use. This is really about creating a new pattern of noticing what you're inclined to do naturally, then consciously making healthier decisions.

The Architecture of Change

The way we behave in any given situation is a choice we make, based on many competing influences. Consciously or not, we tend to weigh the pros and cons of available choices and settle on a particular pattern of behavior, whether it has to do with our eating, drinking, sleeping, exercise, or stress management habits. To change to a new pattern of behavior requires that we, at least partially, abandon the pattern we chose in the first place. Making the switch is difficult, because any change requires giving up the familiar, and the familiar is generally preferred to the unfamiliar. It is certainly easier to stick with the status quo—but remember: Eventually the unfamiliar will become the new familiar.

Starting something new rarely occurs along the path of least resistance. Just as getting a heavy object to start moving across the floor is more difficult than keeping it moving, initiating change is tough. Your priorities are an important part of the equation, since the dietary and activity patterns you have chosen in the past reflect something about the way you presumably want to live. This doesn't mean changing the patterns is impossible, but it does mean it's not as simple as you might hope. It requires preparation and perseverance. It also requires giving your body and brain the support they need—with sufficient sleep, relaxation, and essential nutrients—to bolster your physical and mental fortitude for the challenges that lie ahead.

Even though New Year's resolutions are typically made at the same time of year, there's no reason to think all people are comparably ready to make lasting changes to their behavior at the same time. From the science of behavior modification, the well-known "stages of change," or the transtheoretical model, which was developed by James O. Prochaska, PhD, of the University of Rhode Island, and his colleagues, makes it abundantly clear that when it comes to changing behavior, some people are ready, some are set, and some are already going. But others simply aren't even close to the starting line. If you're in the last camp, the challenge is to begin to get ready by stacking the deck in favor of making changes that will improve your health, your life, and your longevity. But first it helps to recognize where you are now—whether you're contemplating making a change, preparing for it, in the midst of doing it, trying to maintain changes you've made, or struggling to recover from lapses in behavior.

Thomas Edison famously said that "genius is one percent inspiration and ninety-nine percent perspiration." The same is true about making lasting lifestyle changes. Experts in behavior modification generally acknowledge that diet is particularly difficult to change. While smoking cessation is hard to do as well, the decision itself is simple: Yes, you're going to quit, or no, you won't. Physical activity is a little more complicated than that, but not by much. Diet, of course, does not allow for a yes-or-no approach. Food is essential for survival and it cannot be avoided; yet, it imposes considerable risks as well. Unfortunately, when people try to change their behavior in an effort to improve their health and well-being, they often ignore the barriers that stand in their way of making that change. The trouble is, if your schedule makes it difficult to incorporate regular exercise in your life, this obstacle may overcome your motivation to be physically active. Meanwhile, being constantly surrounded by the convenience and familiarity of fast food, while not knowing how to change the way you shop for and prepare healthier meals, can overcome your desire to improve your diet. That's why skillpower is so essential.

Over the years, I've had the impression that many of my patients were discouraged by past attempts to change their behavior, particularly behavior related to weight loss. Many people have tried so many times to eat well, get and stay active, control their weight, and improve their health, without being able to achieve lasting success. Little by little, those "failures" chip away at confidence and even hope. This begs the question: What is it that tends to undo a person's resolve to consume mostly nutritious, disease-fighting foods or to exercise regularly? In large measure, it's the overwhelming resistance presented by the "toxic" nutritional, sedentary environment in which we live, where fast food, junk food, and empty liquid calories are ubiquitous, often in abundant portions, and where little movement is required to get through the day. If you've made multiple attempts to change your diet or physical activity pattern, you may give up entirely and lose your self-efficacy, along with your self-esteem.

This process can be terribly disheartening, to which Nancy, a patient I've known for years, can attest. Now in her late sixties, Nancy is intelligent, active, vivacious, and interesting, and a loving wife, mother, grandmother, sister, and friend. Despite her many positive attributes, Nancy tends to sum herself up in just one word: *fat*. Over time, the work we've done together has helped her lose some 30 pounds, a loss she has maintained for years. And while Nancy is now less critical of her weight than she was before, I'm sorry to say that after literally decades of blaming herself for her inability to control her weight, she has been left with some psychological and emotional scars.

Based on my twenty years of clinical practice, I think the weight of shame, blame, and self-recrimination is far heavier than any number of pounds. This burden needs to be set down first; then the pounds are likely to be shed more readily. While I don't believe in blaming someone for his or her weight struggles, I do believe in taking personal responsibility for the solution. In other words, people can share responsibility for the solution without being to blame for the problem. In order to take responsibility, however, people need to be empowered—with both willpower and skillpower. If either is lacking, failure is likely, which leads us back to self-recrimination and a continued downward spiral. For many years, Nancy lacked the appropriate skillpower, which is why her weight continued to be such a potent source of frustration.

If you're already motivated to change your habits, blaming yourself, or being blamed by others, for not yet doing so is like kicking someone who is already down. It generates feelings of failure and erodes motivation. If you want to lose weight, it's important to realize that doing so is actually far less important than giving up the burden of past weight-loss failures. If you've been unable to change your eating or exercise habits in the past, make a conscious effort to let go of the excess baggage of disappointment, self-blame, or shame. You didn't fail; you just didn't have the right skills.

Think of it this way: You wouldn't blame yourself for *failing* to reach the summit of Mount Everest without having mountaineering skills. In the absence of such skills, you'd have no business even trying! Alas, eating well and being active in the modern world require skillpower, too. If you didn't have those skills the last time you tried to change your habits, you really didn't have a chance. So shrug off your past experiences and get the skills you need this time to reach your goals. That way, you can set yourself up to allow the winds of change to carry you in the right direction—toward better health.

In the simple construct of the Pressure System Model, your answers to just two questions will determine whether you need to focus on raising your motivation, overcoming obstacles, or a bit of both. Ask yourself:

1. Am I currently making optimal, health-promoting, disease-proofing use of my feet and fork?

   If your answer is *yes*, congratulations! Close this book and go read something else.

   If your answer is *no*, go to question 2.

2. Am I ready and willing to make better use of my feet and fork now?

   If your answer is *yes, absolutely*, you have the motivation you need, and it's time to move on to overcoming the impediments in your path.

   If your answer is *kind of* or *maybe*, you probably need to bolster your motivation first, and then work on overcoming impediments, using the steps in this book.

   If your answer is *no*, you are not ready to take on the challenge of change yet. In that case, it's best to devote some time first to working through your ambivalence, using the strategies that follow.

Making the Subconscious Conscious

The reality is that most behaviors are selected without a great deal of conscious consideration. Often they're done on autopilot. It's very doubtful, for example, that you have compiled charts and graphs to characterize the relative pros and cons of sleeping less or more, working hard (or not), exercising (or not), or eating one way or another. But you have, in fact, processed those pros and cons subconsciously by comparing the overall utility, or usefulness to you, of one choice versus others.

You probably know, for example, that sleeping eight hours a night is good for your health. But if you sleep less than that, it's because you're willing to give up the health benefits of more sleep for some alternative benefits (or because you have insomnia). Perhaps by sleeping only six hours a night you can be more productive professionally (or at least you think you can), spend more time with your spouse and/or children, or use the time to keep your home orderly. Even if you end up feeling exhausted or irritable because you're skimping on sleep, you may not make the connection—or want to. We human beings tend to be quite good at rationalizing our choices.

As a result of this unconscious analysis, your motivation for making lifestyle choices can go in several directions simultaneously. You can be motivated to quit smoking (because it will be good for your health) and motivated to continue smoking (because you're addicted or it relaxes you) at the same time. You can be motivated to go out and exercise (because it'll be invigorating) and also be motivated to stay on the couch with the remote in hand (because you're comfortable). You can be motivated to kick a junk food habit while still being motivated to maintain such eating patterns, especially when you're under stress.

The actual measure of motivation that's relevant to your efforts to change is called *effective motivation* (EM), which is the net difference between the motivation to change (MC) and the motivation to maintain the status quo (MM). Here's what it looks like, as an equation: EM = MC – MM. To have a high enough level of effective motivation (EM), you need to shore up your motivation for making the change you desire (MC) so that it's considerably higher than your motivation for maintaining the status quo (MM).

It's human nature to feel two ways about something, but people can get stuck in the quicksand of ambivalence for a long time, instead of moving forward toward a goal. Sometimes you have to consciously and intentionally stack the deck in your favor. But first you'll want to get an accurate assessment of what you're dealing with. After all, if you attempt to change a given behavior, particularly one as challenging as your eating habits, without first doing a ruthlessly honest appraisal of your motivation, you may end up disappointed with the results (or lack thereof).

One effective way to measure motivation and gauge your ambivalence is to construct a *decision balance analysis*, in which you list all the anticipated advantages of making a change in one column and the disadvantages of doing so in another column. You can keep it simple or expand the chart to include the advantages of not making a change along with the disadvantages of that particular choice. (An example is shown in Table 2.1.) Make it as specific or general as you'd like, from "giving your diet an overhaul" to "reducing your sodium intake" to "walking for twenty minutes every day."

Table 2.1. A Decision Balance Chart for Changing vs. Maintaining Your Diet

Changing Diet			
ADVANTAGES	I'll lose weight.	**DISADVANTAGES**	It's hard work.
	I'll improve my health.		I'll have to give up some of my favorite sweets and treats.
	I'll have more energy.		I may feel extra hungry.
	I'll look better.		I may feel stressed.
Maintaining Current Diet			
ADVANTAGES	It's easy.	**DISADVANTAGES**	I won't lose weight.
	I can eat my favorite foods.		I won't get healthier.
	I can relieve stress by snacking.		I might end up gaining weight.
			I might get sick and face large doctor's bills.

You can do this for any behavior change you're considering. The exercise is most useful when the change represents a toss-up—when the motivation levels for making a particular change and maintaining the status quo are about the same. Simply by constructing the decision balance analysis and reviewing it, you may find the additional motivation that's needed to move forward. Alternatively, your analysis may lead to the opposite conclusion: that the cold, hard realities favor maintaining the status quo. In that case, the motivation to maintain the status quo (MM) is higher than the motivation to change (MC), causing effective motivation (EM) to be a negative number. When this happens, there are two likely reasons: The first is that your analysis is incomplete. You have left out some of the advantages of making the change or the disadvantages of not changing. The other is that your analysis is correct but it needs to be altered somehow before it will support your decision to change. You can do this by acquiring new skills that make it easier to change, or by learning new information that makes the appeal of making the change even greater. Finding compelling new items to add to the column on the advantages of changing or the disadvantages of maintaining your current diet, or genuinely removing some of the disadvantages of changing or the advantages of maintaining your current diet will lead to a new conclusion. Pretend Table 2.1 as completed is yours: What else could you say to stack the deck in favor of changing your diet? It may take some active thinking to generate sufficient enthusiasm for changing your behavior, but it's worth the effort.

If you can work through your equivocation about making a change and stack the weight of your decision in favor of doing so, you'll essentially be fortifying your resolve and motivation to take the plunge. As you work through your ambivalence, you may have reason to add to or subtract items from your decision balance table. Each time you alter the balance, you will have a clearer and more complete picture of your motivation. The balance that will send you springing into action could take shape right away or it may occur after multiple revisions—either way is fine, because both realities represent part of the natural process of change. The important thing is that you've initiated the process.

There are other useful ways of cultivating and maximizing your motivation for change. You can increase your motivation with positive or negative imaging. *Positive imaging* involves picturing yourself looking or acting a particular way that's appealing, but that currently eludes you, or imagining how your daily life would be different if you attained those goals. *Negative imaging*, of course, is the converse, reflecting undesirable images, scenes from which you would like to distance yourself by making the desired change. If you know people who have suffered the harmful effects of poor dietary choices and/or sedentary behavior (such as obesity or a heart attack) they can serve as reminders of what you are working to avoid.

Modeling involves finding a pattern of behavior that's similar to the one you want to adopt and using it as a template for your own efforts. Identify people in your life who are setting a good example you might want to follow. If you know someone who consumes a healthy diet, is lean and fit, and seems energetic, he or she can serve as a role model who pumps up your motivation. Whatever the area, you can identify and borrow his or her strategies for success.

Reinforcement involves establishing various ways of discouraging undesired behavior and rewarding desired behavior. Link sticking with your new, more healthful dietary pattern for a certain period to a specific reward (such as buying yourself some new clothes or taking a special outing with friends) and you'll help build up motivation to keep up the good work. On the flip side, creating some type of disincentive to lapsing from the desired pattern may help keep you on track as well (or at least prevent a lapse from turning into a collapse). For example, you might cancel an activity you enjoy if you don't stick with your plan to eat a particular way or be physically active. Only you can decide if you respond better to the prospect of reward or punishment, or to a combination of both.

Publicly making a commitment to change your habits also helps increase motivation. This is called *social contracting*. The commitment itself becomes another reason to change and a positive form of reinforcement. Once you're ready to improve your diet in some way or become more physically active, tell a trusted friend or family member about your plans. This social contracting is helpful in its own right, but it also can lead to other forms of motivational support: Your confidants may provide *social support* by offering to assist you in your efforts, giving positive encouragement when you need it most, or even joining you in your quest for better health. By sharing your aspirations and intentions, you may inspire them to make similar changes, at which point you can offer mutual support and encouragement, reinforce one another's motivation, and/or tap into each other's motivations—thus creating a positive ripple effect.

Ultimately, the most powerful formula for getting and staying healthy is to use moderate amounts of willpower with a heaping dose of skillpower. Will is an essential first skill in the required skill set you'll want to develop in order to master your medical destiny—but it's just one of many. As you'll see in subsequent chapters, other skills are needed to help you create, locate, and navigate your own yellow brick road to better health and well-being. Willpower can get you started, but it's skillpower that enables you to stay the course, and cross the finish line.

When Easy Access Goes Too Far

Ironically, the very things that are now causing the worst public health problems used to be solutions. When our ancestors were hungry, being able to obtain larger quantities of tasty food was a good thing. When previous generations were entirely dependent on muscle power to complete daily tasks, gather food, and flee from danger, the advent of labor-saving devices was a major breakthrough. In both instances, we overshot the solutions and turned them into public enemies that threaten our health, our waistlines, and our well-being.

The result is that some elements of our culture that once might have made sense no longer make any sense at all. I consider these cultural anachronisms—developments that are now behind the times and obsolete because circumstances have moved on, making the developments irrelevant. When we shot past the target of having enough to eat and having a tolerable demand for physical activity, and into the realm of having too much food and not enough activity, we turned elements of our culture from sensible to senseless. We created these anachronisms.

During the Stone Age, the mean survival rate of *Homo sapiens* was estimated at roughly twenty years, and the full span of human life expectancy was about forty. Living was relatively healthy; it just didn't last very long. Now we have the opposite scenario: greater life expectancy but living itself is no longer as healthy.

The basic cause of obesity has always been and always will be energy imbalance—namely, consuming too many calories and not expending enough through physical activity. But the source of calories matters, too. Junk foods have many liabilities, some of which you're probably familiar with. They pack lots of calories into small amounts and tend to be metabolized quickly, thereby spiking insulin levels, which favors fat accumulation in the belly and liver; they also stimulate appetite. High levels of sugar, sodium, and/or fat (ingredients abundant in packaged foods) have been scientifically shown to stimulate the opioid, or pleasure, receptors in the brain, the same ones that are responsive to drugs such as morphine. As a result, processed foods that are loaded with these ingredients can quite literally become addictive.

In a world where brain imaging technology, namely in the form of functional magnetic resonance imaging, is being used to determine what flavor combinations provoke the strongest uptick in appetite, willpower alone isn't going to cut it. You need stronger weapons. When Lays said, "Bet you can't eat just one!" in its potato chip commercials, did you know that they had PhDs on board to make sure that was true? That's right: Manufacturers of processed foods have entire staffs devoted to finding the bliss point of fat, sugar, and/or sodium content that will light up the pleasure centers of your brain, giving you an intense desire to consume more of their product. Adding to the problem is the fact that highly processed foods are aggressively marketed to the public and often have packaging that accentuates the positive, nutritionally speaking, and obscures the negative. Naturally, this makes consumers feel better about buying reduced-fat peanut butter or low-fat cookies and distorts their perspective about what they're actually putting into their bodies when they consume these foods.

Thanks in part to the ubiquity of cars, the conveniences of the Internet, drive-throughs, and automated options, our environment now promotes sedentary behavior. Indeed, we as a society have become increasingly dependent on four wheels. In 1969, 48 percent of children walked to school; in 2009, less than 13 percent did, according to research published in the *American Journal of Preventive Medicine*. This represents a steep decline in daily physical activity not only for kids, but perhaps also for the caregivers who would otherwise walk them to school. While convenient, using machines or technology in place of our muscles poses a threat to personal health. Acknowledging this can help you make more informed, conscious choices, especially when you're not so pressed for time.

Meanwhile, for adults, work has become increasingly workless—in the physical sense, that is. A study recently published by PLoS (short for Public Library of Science) informs us that compared with their 1960s counterparts, the average man and woman now expend roughly 142 fewer calories and 124 fewer calories, respectively, per day at work. Given that there are roughly 240 workdays per year, a man burns approximately 34,000 fewer calories in a year than he would have fifty years ago. Using the standard measure of 3,500 calories equaling 1.0 pound of body fat, this loss in calorie expenditure translates to about 9.7 pounds of weight gain—in just one year! Similarly, a woman burning 124 fewer calories per day would gain 8.5 pounds in one year. This alone could account for much of the modern obesity epidemic.

If we want to alter the rather dire chronic disease trends we have created, there are two potential solutions: We can change the world, or we can change ourselves so we don't succumb en masse to its sabotaging forces. In the current environment, the notion that changing our habits will ensue from willpower alone is at best wishful thinking and at worst downright preposterous. As we've seen, willpower is a necessary part of the solution. And, of course, we need a heaping helping of personal responsibility. But we must also be empowered with the requisite skills. Think of it this way: Relying too much on willpower is like trying to deep-sea dive while only holding your breath—impossible! Skillpower, by contrast, is like learning to use scuba gear. In the beginning, it does take some work to learn how, but once you master the skills and tools, you can stay under water—and continue breathing.

Consider a study published in a 2012 issue of the *Journal of the Academy of Nutrition and Dietetics*: Researchers assigned 189 adults who were responsible for food shopping and food preparation in their households either to a nutrition education group that used a nutrient profiling system to rank foods (according to their vitamin, mineral, and other nutrient content, relative to their calorie content) or to a control group that was given general nutrition information. After eight weeks, the participants who learned the nutrient profiling system were better able to identify nutrient-rich foods; they also did more meal planning, consumed more vegetables and fruits, and overall had a better-quality diet than the control group. The reason: They learned specific skills they could use in the grocery store. Similarly, when overweight adults took a twenty-six-week nutrition and exercise program through the YMCA of metropolitan Atlanta, they ate more fruits and vegetables and exercised more frequently, which led to substantial weight loss. Chalk up another win for skillpower!

Given these realities, it's essential to find the course toward healthier living and a healthier future—and to stay on it. To some extent, these efforts will need to defy the influences inherent in our obesigenic environment, but it can be done, and it isn't as difficult as most people think. To start, choosing more foods that come from the earth instead of food factories will set you on the right course toward better health and greater longevity. Seize a variety of opportunities to move your body—whether by taking the stairs instead of the elevator whenever possible, walking on errands instead of driving, or choosing physically active pursuits for your family over sedentary ones. These are choices that require skill-power, not just willpower.

Will and skill are related in ways people tend to overlook. Having the right skillpower makes a task easier, thereby reducing the amount of will-power you will need to get the job done. To illustrate this point, I often think of my medical training. Medical residency (those years of training in a hospital that immediately follow medical school) is notoriously bru-tal, even now that limits have been placed on the number of consecutive hours residents are on duty. When I was a resident, I was at times on call every fourth night; other times every third night. That means I'd go to work on Monday, work all through the day and night, work all day Tues-day, go home on Tuesday night, get up and go to work on Wednesday, then go home that night. Come Thursday, the pattern would repeat. But this was a cakewalk compared to medical training in my dad's day. He was on call every other night: He'd work thirty-six hours or so, go home and sleep, then repeat the pattern—and he did this for years. *Yikes!*

The medical residency experience has gotten better over the years, but it is still pretty harsh, and perhaps with good reason. To make the transition from being a civilian to a doctor who can make life-or-death decisions (and get them right more often than not) under tremendous time pressure and the strains of exhaustion is a big deal. To do what is required during that transition is what I often refer to as "external disci-pline." It's an array of rules, regulations, and routines that *make* you do the right things, that make you *learn* a whole new way of behaving. At first, medical residents simply don't have the internal guidance system to do this, so a system of regulations keeps them on track. There are strict rules, for example, about evaluating a fever, responding to a call from the emer-gency room, admitting a new patient to the hospital, and handling a car-diac arrest. There are requirements about when to draw blood and check lab results, when to make rounds, and when to fill out charts. By the time doctors come through this grueling experience, something truly remark-able happens: We have internalized all those rules. In fact, what started out being all about rules ends up being all about habit, even instinct.

There's a lesson here. If you want to change your habits, one approach is to try really, really hard; this is one version of willpower. The other is to follow the rules until that external discipline becomes internal discipline; that's how skillpower is developed. The rules relieve the burden on your willpower, and once you have internalized them, they become part of your personal skill set, resulting in a positive chain reaction.

Closer to home is the example of going on a diet. For the most part, diets fail to produce long-term weight loss. They work in the short term because of rules about what and when you can and can't eat: They prevent you from going off-course with external discipline. That's why it doesn't really matter (in terms of short-term weight loss) if you cut fat or carbs, eat only bacon or Twinkies, eat only under the light of a full moon or while standing on one foot, or do any other wacky thing. What matters is that if you go from undisciplined eating to disciplined eating, even if the discipline in question is silly and can't be sustained, you will likely lose weight in the short term.

Most diets don't offer a form of discipline you can reasonably internalize. Sure, you can lose weight by eating nothing except bacon in the short term, but you definitely won't improve your eating habits or your health that way in the long term. You will probably also get tired of eating bacon. The kind of discipline that diets provide is meant to be temporary, even though the challenge of weight control is permanent—a situation involving dissonance.

An alternative approach has a vastly greater chance of long-term success: Combine willpower with external discipline until you can develop your own internal skillpower. Yes, the process starts with willpower because you need to *want* to change your weight, your health, and your lifestyle for it to happen. But you'll want to add in some external discipline—not the "go on a diet" kind that you can't stick with over time, but the kind that's used to train doctors, soldiers, pilots, or scuba divers. This kind of discipline includes rules that you can internalize to become part of your mind-set and your standard operating procedure forever.

Once that happens, you will come to rely on skillpower more, and find that willpower is much, much less important.

So, after you've taken steps to assess your willpower, maximize your motivation, and work through your ambivalence, it's time to apply some external discipline to help you achieve your goals. Besides lightening the burden on your willpower, this will buy you sufficient time to develop the skillpower that will allow you to make desired lifestyle changes for good. In Table 2.2, you'll find a set of "rules" that will help you start losing excess weight, increasing your fitness level, and improving your overall health. These are guidelines you can follow forever, or until they become a regular part of your life. For them to work, though, you have to be consistent. This is not an on-again, off-again proposition, but the rewards to your health will be worth it. Following these maxims is essentially the first step toward living more healthfully.

Table 2.2. The Ten Rules of External Discipline (TRED) for Healthy Living

Rule	Purpose
1. Avoid fast food	Fast food is a fast pass to weight gain and health problems. Avoid it while you initiate a lifestyle makeover. It's too late once you're at the drive-through asking, "Should I or shouldn't I?" If, for some reason, you can't avoid fast-food restaurants, use www.healthydiningfinder.com to upgrade your choices.
2. Drink water	Liquid calories don't usually fill you up, but they can certainly add up. Soft drinks, juices, and the like are very sugary, encouraging your sweet tooth to grow into a sweet fang. Put soda out of bounds; when you're thirsty, drink water (dressed up with lemon, lime, or orange slices, if preferred). Steer clear of diet soda, except as a brief transition from regular soda to something truly wholesome such as water. Artificial sweeteners in diet soda propagate a sweet tooth, and the sugar/calories you've saved tend to sneak back in elsewhere.

(continued)

Rule	Purpose
3. Eat salad	Mixed greens are loaded with nutrients and have almost no calories. Including a mixed green salad—with just a tablespoon or two of dressing (or olive oil and vinegar)—at the start of every dinner will help fill you up so you eat fewer calories overall.
4. Get some exercise every day	As you start your health makeover, you should get moving. Begin with at least twenty minutes of any form of exercise, as intense as walking briskly, no fewer than five days a week. Make it a rule and honor it.
5. Make sleep a priority	If you sleep enough and soundly, you will have more control over your appetite and more energy for exercise. Commit to a consistent eight hours per night if at all possible; use good sleep hygiene (see chapter 12) to help you stay on course.
6. Mind your mouth	Avoid mindless eating. Eat only when eating is your primary activity; don't munch while you're doing something else. It's easy to eat too much or the wrong foods that way without realizing it (often referred to as eating amnesia).
7. Eat foods with identifiable ingredients	Avoid foods that contain ingredients an eight-year-old can't pronounce. Otherwise, you may end up consuming a mouthful of additives and chemicals that offer little or no nutritional value. With real food, you can tell what the ingredients are; with manufactured foods, you often can't.
8. Plan all eating occasions	Go off the "see food" diet. Eat only what you intended to eat, when you intended to eat it. Don't eat just because food—say, a slice of cake at an office birthday party—is there. Eat when you're hungry and stop when you've had enough—*before* you're truly full.

(continued)

Rule	Purpose
9. Tell everyone	Tell the most important people in your life what health-related changes you want to make and why. And tell them about these rules so they can help you stick to them.
10. Choose what you chew*	Take control of your choices, both at home and when you're out. Use an insulated snack pack to take wholesome foods wherever you go, so you always have them at your fingertips. See chapter 9 for suggestions.

*A shout-out of thanks to Kellee McQuinn, of kidtribe.com, for this great line, penned as lyrics for the music video "Unjunk Yourself!" (http://www.youtube.com /watch?v=PLaS0En9Q98).

Getting the Right Power Alignment

The importance of aligning skillpower with willpower is nicely illustrated by another important behavioral choice: the decision to quit smoking. Quite a few years ago, I was thinking about why so many people who *tried* to quit smoking *failed* to quit smoking. Clearly, they were motivated; otherwise, they wouldn't be trying to kick the habit. It might, of course, be the obvious: nicotine addiction. But even people who try to quit smoking with nicotine replacement therapy and/or prescription drugs often fail. So what accounts for this? It occurred to me that there might be barriers to quitting that were flying under the radar and not being addressed.

To get to the bottom of it, I thought of this metaphor: Imagine there is a prize, such as a large pot of gold, on the far side of a field, and you *really* want to get there. But, alas, there is a high stone wall in the way, without windows or a door, and there's no way around it. It seemed to me that trying to quit smoking on your own—with the pot of gold being better health—might feel this way. Now imagine that your doctor comes along and offers help that's equivalent to the form of a wrecking ball that could knock a big hole through the wall. Suddenly you might feel it's easy to get to the pot of gold. But what if behind the first wall, there were another wall, and then another wall after that, and so on?

When I thought about the challenge of smoking cessation this way, I wondered, how many walls are there really between a person's intention or will to quit and the goal of being smoke-free? Is there a finite list of impediments that commonly cause attempts to quit smoking to fail? As it turns out, the answer is a decisive yes. There are, in fact, seven common reasons that people who want to quit smoking fail to do so. They are nicotine addiction, anxiety and/or depression, alcoholism, another chemical dependency, stress, living with another smoker, and fear of weight gain. Some aspiring quitters face all these obstacles, others have a few, and most have more than just one. If you think of each barrier as a stone wall, suddenly it's quite obvious why people who want to quit smoking, and who even get help to do so, still fail. It's not enough to have a wrecking ball to knock down some of the walls; unless they all come tumbling down, you still won't succeed.

After I posed the question about what stands between people and succeeding at changing their health-related behavior, my colleagues and I developed a behavior modification technique called *impediment profiling*. Over the years, we have conducted and published a number of studies using this method—and we have found that it works. What my colleagues and I did was establish an impediment profiler for smoking cessation that helped reveal which of the seven barriers any individual had. We then tailored treatments accordingly, at times providing an individual with ways to address all seven impediments. The result, in a series of pilot studies, was unprecedented quit rates. The majority of smokers who participated in the studies quit, and half were still successful a year later; these results are twice as good as with the usual approaches.

The idea behind impediment profiling is relevant to other lifestyle changes. In a study involving 1,687 young adults, researchers at the University of Minnesota found that the majority enjoyed and valued eating with other people, and those who regularly ate dinner with others had a better overall diet, including a higher intake of fruit and vegetables; yet 35 percent of the men and 42 percent of the women reported having trouble finding time to sit down for a meal with other people. That's an impediment that involves time constraints and planning, among other factors. If these young adults could find ways around those obstacles, they'd improve the quality of their diet and their enjoyment of meals and create more opportunities for social connection, too—a triple win. But a change like that takes skillpower.

If you can identify what's stopping you from improving your eating habits or incorporating more movement in your life, you can develop skills that will help you surmount those obstacles. Problem solving or troubleshooting is an essential part of the picture. In a study involving 272 women participating in a six-month lifestyle intervention designed to help them lose weight, researchers at the University of Florida, Gainesville, found that those who improved their problem-solving abilities—by setting weekly goals for altering their eating and exercising behavior, anticipating obstacles, and strategizing possible solutions—lost more weight (more than 10 percent of their body weight) and stuck to the program better than those who didn't.

There are many different skills that can help you reach the brass ring. You can enhance your awareness of what causes you to overeat and adjust your environment to favor moderation. You can use the volume of food you choose to help you fill up on fewer calories. You can learn how to interpret food labels and how to avoid an excessive variety of flavors in any given meal or snack (since flavor overload can coax you to eat more). The more skills you acquire by reading and heeding the following chapters, the better prepared you will be for any situation. There are vital skills related to shopping and cooking, managing time, and fitting exercise into an already hectic daily routine. For every challenge your environment throws in the path to better health, there is a relevant skill to help you get over or around it. You'll build an entire tool kit that will allow you to reach or maintain a healthy weight, get or stay fit, and fight diseases before they start. It could quite possibly save your life.

• Three •

The Heave-Ho Prescription

Contrary to the oft-quoted aphorism, knowledge isn't quite power; it's more of a prerequisite for power. Real power depends on being able to put what you know to work. In the case of healthful living and disease prevention, knowledge is a necessity for cultivating the will to forge a path to a healthier lifestyle and future. The challenge, of course, is to care deeply and passionately enough to turn what you know into a routine. You don't have to be perfect in your actions; rather, the goal is to focus on making steady progress toward improving your diet and becoming more physically active. You may or may not reach your ideal weight by making these changes, but you will certainly move toward it, and more important, you will improve your health, which is actually the ultimate aim.

As it turns out, we are all making life-or-death decisions every single day in terms of what we choose to put into our bodies and how we choose to use them. So why not choose the positive path that will lead you toward greater health and longevity? Archimedes said, "Give me a lever long enough and . . . I can single handed[ly] move the world." Well, the levers to move your health to a better place are indeed long enough for the job—and they are in your hands. The knowledge and power to use them should be, too.

With those levers, you can reach all the way into the double helix of your DNA—and make even your genes healthier. One of the eye-opening revelations provided by the Human Genome Project, which was completed in 2003, is that genes by themselves don't lead to disease. It's the interaction of certain high-risk genes and unhealthy environmental influences (including poor diet, physical inactivity, and smoking) that combine to trigger diseases.

The goal, then, is to use your feet, forks, and fingers wisely for the sake of your health—so you can move those levers in the right direction and improve your future. It's not at all complicated; it's just unfamiliar. You don't have to lead a Spartan, monastic existence or live on Planet Health. The key is to learn to love foods that will love you back, to seize as many opportunities as possible to move your body, and to refrain from (or quit) damaging habits such as smoking. These are the tools and habits you need to use wisely to live healthfully on this planet.

Consider a day in the life of you and your fork: You'll have choices to make for breakfast, lunch, dinner, and snacks. At work, you may have to decide whether to take something from the tray of donuts or bagels in the conference room or whether to grab a handful of jelly beans from your colleague's ever-present (and always full) candy jar. You may have to decide between joining your coworkers as they head to a fast-food joint for lunch or taking a healthier route on your own. And if you go out to dinner, you'll face a smorgasbord of choices, far more than you would have from the relatively limited options in your own kitchen.

Similarly, you and your feet will have numerous chances to coordinate your efforts, whether it's for a workout at the time of your choosing, walking your children to and from school or the bus, or hoofing it on errands. You'll have many opportunities to decide whether to take the stairs or elevator in an office building or to e-mail a colleague rather than walk over to her desk. After work and on the weekends, you'll have decisions to make about how to engage in pleasant activities with family members or friends—including whether to make those activities physical and what you'll eat.

Each of these opportunities will present its own set of challenges, which is why moving toward better health is really a skill-dependent enterprise. Of course, we all wish it were easy and automatic to live healthfully and avoid chronic diseases. But if it were . . . well, we'd have a few bridges to sell you! The truth is that there's only practical magic, which involves mastering the right skill set to move you toward a state of better health and well-being. During the course of any given day, you can make health-promoting decisions that involve food or physical activity. As already noted, the right food choices and physical activities can protect you from dreaded chronic diseases that may lead to premature death or disability. Want proof? Consider this: In a study involving 713 women in their seventies, researchers at the University of Michigan and the National Institute on Aging found that the women who were the most physically active had a 72 percent lower mortality rate over five years than their sedentary peers. Those with the highest fruit and vegetable consumption (as measured by blood levels of carotenoids, a class of health-promoting plant pigments) were 50 percent more likely to survive the five-year follow-up period than women with the lowest fruit and vegetable intake.

To some extent, efforts to improve your diet and physical activity patterns will need to defy the influences that are inherent in our obesity-promoting environment. But it can be done, and it isn't as difficult as people think it is. And once you begin to reap the rewards of eating well and moving more, the fruits of your efforts will serve as positive reinforcement for continuing the good work you have undertaken. After all, gaining skillpower can be inherently empowering. Just as it's gratifying and enjoyable to master a new skill (such as playing the piano or cooking paella), a new sport (such as learning to ski), or a new talent (such as developing the fancy footwork that enables you to dance gracefully), it can be satisfying and heartening to learn how to live more healthfully. And the potential payoff really is tremendous: Refashioning your medical destiny at the genetic level, enhancing the way you feel and function in everyday life, and bestowing the gift of healthy habits and less illness on your loved ones. Think of it as a prescription for what we all need to know and do to make things right, health-wise, in our current environment.

Proof that we need this mandate: As mentioned earlier, improvements in lifestyle can lead to an 80 percent reduction in heart disease, a 90 percent reduction in diabetes, and a 60 percent drop in cancer rates.

Moreover, research has found that people are 80 percent less likely to get any major chronic disease if they have the right answers to the following four questions: Do you smoke? Do you eat well? Do you get regular physical activity? Do you control your weight?

Let's consider these elements one by one. It's widely known that smoking is a potent risk factor for lung cancer, heart disease, and stroke. But the fact is, the habit also has been linked with cancers of the mouth, throat, voice box, breast, stomach, bladder, cervix, uterus, and kidneys. Smoking is also associated with infertility, osteoporosis, preterm delivery and low birth weight, emphysema, and bronchitis. According to the Centers for Disease Control and Prevention, tobacco use causes more deaths each year than "all deaths from human immunodeficiency virus (HIV), illegal drug use, alcohol use, motor vehicle injuries, suicides, and murders combined." That's right: *Combined*. That's why it's smart to abstain from smoking altogether. If you do smoke, quit—it's as simple as that. You'll breathe easier and live longer and more healthfully.

An optimal diet (a prudent use of forks) also exerts far-ranging, positive effects on every aspect of physiology—from enhancing your energy, immune function, digestion, bone health, and physical performance to improving your mood and various aspects of cognitive (mental) function. A healthy diet that's loaded with fruits, vegetables, whole grains, beans, legumes, nuts, seeds, low-fat or nonfat dairy foods, and moderate amounts of lean protein stands to reduce the risk of chronic conditions such as heart disease, hypertension, cholesterol abnormalities, cancer, osteoporosis, and diabetes. Simply put, a healthy diet provides your body with the nutrients it needs to perform everyday functions, preserve wellness, and fight disease. In a sense, food really can be powerful medicine—and so can movement.

After all, regular physical activity (an excellent use of your feet) is associated with reduced inflammation throughout your body, improved immune function, better circulation and heart health, greater bone density and muscle strength, and greater overall quality of life. Fitness that stems from regular physical activity reduces the risk of diabetes, heart disease, stroke, cancer, and disabling arthritis, among other diseases. Being physically active on a daily basis also enhances concentration, memory, and productivity.

On the subject of body weight, it's important to note that weight is not a behavior. But it is controlled (partly) by behaviors. There are, to be sure, important genetic influences—you are not totally in control of your weight. But to the extent that you are—and for most of us, that's a very large extent—it's a simple proposition that's governed primarily by calories in (from foods and beverages) versus calories out (those that are expended through physical activity). Simple doesn't mean easy, of course! Controlling weight in this modern world is hard; in fact, most people don't manage it. But hard doesn't mean complicated. Lifting a heavy rock is hard but it's not complicated. The same is true of setting down the extra weight you wish you weren't carrying.

Achieving the best balance that you can in the current world is a personal responsibility, for the simple reason that nobody else will do it for you. People who gain excess weight over time are in a state of what's called a positive energy balance, which is not a good thing. The longer that state persists, and the greater the imbalance is, the more weight that is gained.

In research conducted from my lab at Yale, my colleagues and I have identified the most common impediments and obstacles people encounter when trying to improve their diet and exercise habits. Across various demographic profiles, the patterns are similar. When it comes to making better dietary choices, people of various ages and socioeconomic levels often face dozens of barriers, including not knowing what a healthy diet looks like or how to shop for or cook healthy foods; struggling with time constraints and hectic schedules; eating for emotional reasons; and dealing with picky eaters in the family. The same is true on the physical activity front: Across many ages and stages of life, common barriers include lack of knowledge about how to begin an exercise regimen, time and scheduling challenges, lack of social support, insufficient motivation or energy, and financial limitations.

Besides identifying common ground in terms of what's stopping people from improving their lifestyles, my research team has devised strategies for helping people overcome these barriers—and we have proven that they work. We found that when we provided strategies, resources, and expert advice that would help people deal with their personal barriers to being more physically active, their physical activity rates picked up significantly. Similarly, when we gave people the skills and strategies they needed, they were able to make healthy dietary changes. If you consider *all* the potential barriers and identify those that affect you, you can work to acquire a helpful strategy, skill, or tool that will get you past that barrier, and then the barrier will no longer be a barrier. What's more, you'll have successfully made a change. When you have done this for every barrier you face and developed habits that will protect your health and fight diseases, you will have gained power over your lifestyle. You will have mastered the means to get over, around, or through the barriers so that you can attain better health.

In the chapters that follow, you will learn the comprehensive set of skills that will help you bust through your obstacles and come out the other side—into the domains of greater wellness and vitality. You will find a detailed, step-by-step guide to acquiring the relevant skills and using them in a way that will allow you to take charge of the levers that influence your medical future. This isn't a plan exclusively to prevent heart disease. It's not a plan simply to avoid cancer. And it's not just a plan to dodge diabetes. It's an approach that will help you do all of that—and more!—because it's an all-inclusive set of life-saving skills. Think of this as one-stop shopping for living more healthfully and happily and living longer—the ultimate prizes.

I used to teach a course at the Yale School of Public Health called Clinical Concepts in Public Health, for students who were getting their master's degrees in public health. It was, in essence, medical school's greatest hits—everything fascinating about how the body works and fails—condensed into a single semester. The challenge with teaching the course, which I divided up by organ systems (e.g., the cardiovascular system, the nervous system, the respiratory system), was that the anklebone really *is* connected to the shinbone (and the cardiovascular system is connected to the respiratory system, etc.). In other words, you can't fully understand the heart without understanding the lungs and kidneys, too. You can't understand the kidneys without understanding the endocrine system (hormones) and the nervous system. You can't understand the nervous system . . . and so on.

The only solution was to teach one organ system at a time, while referring to the others as needed. Otherwise, I would have had to interrupt a lecture on the cardiovascular system with a lecture on the genitourinary system and then in turn interrupt that lecture to cover some other system. It would have been confusing at best, chaotic at worst. So I kept cross-referencing material as we went through the curriculum, and frequently encouraged the students to "wait for it!" That's how we rolled—and it worked.

This approach works with the skills for healthy living, too, because these skills really are as interconnected and interdependent as different organ systems in the body. This reality makes it hard to talk about them in isolation, but just as the organ systems in the body come together to create one harmonious product—namely, you!—so do the skills that can guide your health in a more positive direction. That's the power and beauty of what I call *skill synergy*. The skills for living healthfully are interrelated, and each one you learn makes it easier to learn and apply the next.

In the following chapters, you'll learn about the specific skills that will help you improve your eating and movement habits. As you continue through the book, identify the skills and sections that are most relevant to you, so that you can begin to develop your own customized plan of action. (If you want to take a shortcut to identify the skills you need to develop most, you can use the Skill Spiral, a personalized approach that will help you take steps to better health, in chapter 12.) By acquiring skills in the most logical sequence for you, you can use each one to make the next one easier, and in the process rise a bit higher toward your goal of disease-proof vitality.

The accumulation of these disease-fighting skills will culminate in true mastery, allowing you to better steer yourself and your family to-

ward a healthier future and perhaps a longer one, too. You will be fortifying your health from the helical spiral of your DNA on out. Improve the
way you use your feet and forks, in particular, and you may be able to
alter the expression of genes that make you vulnerable to developing a
particular disease, even after you've been diagnosed with a disease. Each
of us already holds the power to change the course of our health trajectory. It's time to exercise that power by exerting the all-important heave-
ho on that mighty lever.

A Day in the Life of You and Your Fork

Over the course of any given day, there are many opportunities for you
to eat well—or badly. By looking across the expanse of that prototypical
day, you can see that each time you and food come together, good or bad
things can happen, depending on the skill set you bring with you into the
encounter. Table 3.1 addresses how to get through every conceivable eating occasion that may (or may not) occur, while maintaining optimal
nutrition. For each such occasion, there's an approach and a set of skills
that are essential to making it a healthy eating experience. (The chapters
that follow address these skills in detail.)

Table 3.1. A Day in the Life of You and Your Fork

Eating occasion	Optimal eating depends on	Which, in turn, depends on
A.M./breakfast	Having nutritious ingredients readily available for a healthy breakfast	• Identifying and buying nutritious foods • Being motivated to choose nutritious foods • Having the skills to know how to assemble foods quickly and conveniently into a nutritious meal

(continued)

Eating occasion	Optimal eating depends on	Which, in turn, depends on
A.M. snack	Having nutritious foods on hand for a quick, convenient, satiating snack wherever you are	• Having nutritious foods at home • Being able to identify and choose foods that are satisfying and filling and that travel well
P.M./lunch	Having a nutritious lunch	• Same as for A.M./breakfast • Being able to identify and choose a wholesome lunch away from home
P.M. snack	Having a nutritious and satisfying afternoon snack on hand	• Same as for A.M. snack • Being able to find, choose, and buy a wholesome snack outside the home
Dinner, home	Having a nutritious, satisfying, family-friendly, convenient dinner	• Same as for breakfast and lunch • Having the skills to cook wholesome meals • Being able to communicate with family members about the importance of healthful eating and engage them in it • Establishing an inventory of food choices that are satisfactory to all

(continued)

Eating occasion	Optimal eating depends on	Which, in turn, depends on
Dinner, out	Having a nutritious and satisfying restaurant meal	• Knowing which restaurants are healthier than others • Knowing how to identify the best options on any menu • Knowing what questions to pose to the server and/or chef • Knowing how to identify proper portion sizes
Drinking	Choosing water most times and the best possible alternatives at other times	• Knowing what beverages are best and having them available
Traveling	Maintaining a healthful dietary pattern while traveling	• Being prepared to take nutritious foods with you on the road • Knowing how to identify the best choices when eating out
General/Other	Recognizing and overcoming emotional reasons for eating	• Being able to troubleshoot mindless or emotional eating • Being able to prevent or manage cravings

A Day in the Life of You and Your Feet

Over the course of any given day, there are many opportunities for you to be active or sedentary. By looking across the expanse of a prototypical day in the life of you and your feet, you'll see that each situation presents an opportunity for activity of some kind, and each opportunity depends on a particular application of skillpower. Table 3.2 addresses how to fit physical activity into your daily routine—no matter what. For each occasion, there's an approach and a set of skills that are essential to making physical activity happen. (Chapters 10 and 11 address these skills in detail.)

Table 3.2. A Day in the Life of You and Your Feet

Situation	Optimal activity depends on	Which, in turn, depends on
A.M.	Fitting in a morning workout	• Being motivated to exercise • Having a workout routine (and a place to do it) planned
Workday	Fitting physical activity into the workday's activities	• Having an activity option that suits the work venue and schedule • Taking stairs instead of elevators • Walking to nearby errands instead of driving
Your child's school day	Creating opportunities for movement during the school day	• Having an activity option that suits the school venue and schedule • Being able to include short bouts of movement into the day's activities

(continued)

Situation	Optimal activity depends on	Which, in turn, depends on
Leisure day	Making physical activity part of a day of leisure/recreation	• Enjoying physically active hobbies and outings • Having physically active options suitable for enjoyment/recreation • Making exercise social
Travel	Fitting physical activity in when on the road	• Having an arsenal of exercises that can be done in brief bursts wherever you are • Knowing how to customize physical activity to suit any location • Being able to manage your time well
P.M.	Fitting in an evening workout	• Same as the A.M.
Vacation and family time	Making physically active recreation part of a personal or family vacation Engaging in physical activity with other family members	• Same as leisure day • Communicating with family members about the importance of physical activity • Being able to combine physical activity with family recreation • Walking places with your family instead of driving

• Four •

Developing Nutritional Knowledge—and Power

The Challenge: You can't eat healthfully if you don't know what healthy eating looks like.

The Right Response: Get an authoritative overview of good nutrition from a source you can trust—namely, this book.

The Relevant Skills: Identifying the fundamentals of good nutrition; reshaping your plate; exercising portion control; putting fullness (satiety) on your side; and thinking about your drinks.

Just as you wouldn't ordinarily set off on a trip without knowing where your destination was, you can't embark on the challenge of eating more healthfully without knowing what that entails. You need to know where you're going—in this case, what a healthy diet actually looks like—before you can get there. Otherwise, how can you possibly make wholesome choices for how you use your fork throughout the day? Once you know what constitutes a healthy diet, you'll be able to develop the skillpower that will allow you to translate that knowledge into effective action.

Still, doing so can be a confusing proposition, given all the conflicting nutritional advice that's out there. On the one hand, Dr. Robert Lustig, from the University of California, San Francisco, tells us that sugar is dietary evil number one, while the Center for Science in the

Public Interest, an advocacy group based in Washington, D.C., points its collective finger at salt as being a singularly dangerous dietary culprit. Biochemist T. Colin Campbell, of Cornell University, attributes our health woes to animal protein, and Dr. Caldwell Esselstyn, of the Cleveland Clinic, says lecithin, a fatty substance in animal tissues and some plants, is to blame. Meanwhile, Dr. Dean Ornish, founder of the Preventive Medicine Research Institute, says that a low-fat, plant-based diet is the answer to many of our country's health problems, whereas a fairly radical contingent of advocates for our Stone Age diet argues for the important benefits of eating meat. Then there are the purists, many of whom claim that eating raw foods that come directly from nature is the only way to go. They can't all be right! So whom should we believe?

There's a kernel of truth in most, if not all, of these claims. People get very zealous about a particular approach to diet. But just as with religion, others with comparable credentials and fervor make a completely different case. The mingling of religious-style zealotry and opinions about nutrition principles is a growing but ominous trend—and it often steers people off course from what truly matters. So while many of these ideas deserve a place at the table, none of them should be the only one sitting there. Yes, consuming too much sugar is bad for you. It tends to travel in high-calorie foods (which can also promote weight gain), and it creates a desire for more sugary foods (ditto). Too much salt in the diet can promote high blood pressure and make you crave more salt, perpetuating a less-than-healthy eating style. Consuming animal protein isn't necessarily a problem, unless you eat too much of it and it's loaded with fat.

The basics of what constitutes a healthy diet are well established, and they represent the overlap of almost every *good* diet with one another; however, there is room for variation on the theme of healthy eating, which is good, because it gives each of us options and puts us in the driver's seat. It would be great if more of our foods came directly from the field to plate, but in the real world, people, even healthy people, occasionally eat a chip or another food that comes in a bag, box, bottle, jar, or can. This can be bad, but it isn't always. When it comes to packaged foods, it's hard to indict pure almond butter (in a jar), dried lentils (in a bag), or a box of raisins. And pure tomato paste (in a can) hardly qualifies as a food felony. We have considerable evidence that better choices can be made among packaged foods, and that making those better choices can help promote better health. I recently heard about a mom who lost 115 pounds, thanks almost entirely to her use of the NuVal System, a nutrition guidance program that a team of scientists and I developed that scores foods on a scale from 1 to 100 (the higher the number, the more nutritious the food). Using NuVal Scores helped her trade up to more nutritious choices in every aisle of her supermarket, and by addressing the quality of what she ate, and what she served her family, the issues of quantity and weight-control efforts mostly took care of themselves. (In chapter 7, you'll learn more about the NuVal System and how to use it for your own benefit.)

In Search of the Ideal Diet

There's no real mystery about what's required for the basic care and feeding of humans. Despite evolution and technological advances over the centuries, and despite the health information whiplash caused by the media, the dietary approach that supports health and wellness for humans today is not all that different from what did it for our ancestors. Before delving into the details, let's consider a question that addresses this at the most commonsensical level: If you were a zookeeper, and you were getting some koala bears to care for, how would you decide what to feed them? Would you: (a) consult the author of a fad diet book; (b) run a randomized, double-blind, controlled trial; or (c) feed them something like what they were eating in the wild? The obvious answer, and the approach that actually is used by zoos and wildlife specialists all over the world, is option *c*. We don't run clinical trials to see how koala bears fare on a diet consisting of hunks of wildebeest or platters of eucalyptus leaves, and, well, the market for fad diet books for koalas is mighty slim.

So while it may not answer every question or solve every potential health problem, the optimal starting point for knowing what creatures ought to eat is: their native diet.

Human beings are no exception in this respect. We, too, have a native diet. The experts who are best suited to tell us what that diet is are called paleoanthropologists—that is, anthropologists specializing in the Stone Age, which represents the vast majority of human history. Of course, no one can say exactly what people ate every day tens of thousands of years ago. It's tough enough to remember exactly what we had for breakfast yesterday. But by studying fossilized human waste and patterns of dental wear, and by knowing what foods were available at the time, the paleoanthropologists have put together a pretty good mosaic of what our native diet and lifestyle probably looked like. Some aspects are quite obvious: Our Stone Age ancestors ate foods that came directly from nature; they didn't eat processed foods, because the manufacturing of food simply had not been invented.

Approximately half the calories in the Stone Age diet are thought to have come from plants, the other half from meat. Plant foods are far less concentrated in calories than animal foods are. To have derived half of one's calories from plant foods meant eating a lot more plant foods, in terms of mass or volume, than animal foods. Remember, too, that modern meat is not the same as Stone Age meat. The animal meat our ancestors ate was generally quite lean, often with fat content around 10 percent of calories per serving, sometimes lower. Back then, there were no slop-fed pigs, no grain-fed cattle, and no domesticated feed animals that were raised without physical challenges to their muscles. The fat in their meat also was far more unsaturated than the fat in most modern meats (because the animals ate a rich variety of wild plant foods and were active) and even provided some omega-3 fatty acids (which are necessary for human health but can't be manufactured by the body). Back then, there was no such thing as corned beef, salami, pastrami, hot dogs, or hamburgers—processed meat was certainly not on the Paleo diet. (In modern times, the flesh of antelope, grass-fed cattle, and bison best approximates the Paleo experience.)

From the *Things-You-Never-Knew-You-Never-Knew* Files

Experts suggest that our Paleolithic ancestors consumed as much as 100 grams of fiber per day, from a variety of plant foods eaten in large enough quantities to fuel that high demand for physical energy. We know they did a lot of walking—but they must have stopped to squat pretty often!

Based on common sense, an understanding of our native diet, and a very large volume of convergent modern science, we have a compelling case for eating mostly plants for reasons related to both our health and weight. Generally, plant foods are a far more concentrated source of vitamins and minerals and a much less concentrated source of calories and fat than animal foods. In summarizing an essential rule for healthy living in his book *In Defense of Food: An Eater's Manifesto*, Michael Pollan advises simply but eloquently, "Eat food. Not too much. Mostly plants." My personal belief is this is excellent advice, but there are variations on the principles of healthful eating—which is good, because this leaves us with options. It puts each of us in the driver's seat, where we belong, and maximizes the opportunities for us to love foods that will love us back—nutritious and delicious foods that appeal to our senses but also help our bodies run well, stay strong, build vitality, and so on.

People often ask me, "What's the best diet?" Last year, a woman named Elizabeth came to see me for this very reason. She had recently gone through menopause, wanted to lose belly fat (and avoid joining family members suffering from diabetes and heart disease), and needed to sort through conflicting nutritional advice she'd received about how to do it. Elizabeth's personal trainer, with whom she exercises five days a week, had been advising her to eat more frequently throughout the day and to include protein supplements to keep her metabolic fires stoked. Meanwhile, a nutritionist she consulted had recommended that Elizabeth space out her meals further, to help her cut her overall calorie con-

sumption and lose those extra 15 pounds. I told her that having a rigid
zeal about either approach is unfounded. If it works for someone to eat
six mini-meals instead of three square meals a day, or vice versa, there's
no problem with that, as long as it's done in a reasonable fashion, in
terms of the meal's content and portion sizes.

The fact is that healthful eating consistently emphasizes the same
foods: vegetables, fruits, beans, legumes, nuts, seeds, and whole grains.
Some variations (such as the Mediterranean diet) include fish and seafood; others (such as the vegan diet) do not. Some (such as the Dietary
Approaches to Stop Hypertension, or DASH diet, and the diet used in
the Diabetes Prevention Program) include low- and nonfat dairy; others
do not. Some (such as the Mediterranean, Paleo, South Beach, Sonoma,
and DASH diets) include lean meats; others (such as Dr. Dean Ornish's
plan and the raw foods diet) do not. And some (such as the Portfolio
Diet) contain large amounts of fiber. All banish highly processed foods
that deliver concentrated doses of refined starch, sugar, trans fats, certain
saturated fats, and/or salt.

Whatever approach it takes, the "best" diet must be sustainable. It
can't be just about losing weight; it has to be just as much about finding,
gaining, and maintaining health. There are many different ways to get
there. Research from Laval University, in Quebec, found that two different diet approaches—one that restricted fat intake and one that emphasized including more fruits and vegetables—both led to similar weight
loss results among overweight women after one year. More recently, researchers from the New Balance Foundation Obesity Prevention Center,
Boston Children's Hospital, compared the effects of a low-fat diet, a very-
low-carbohydrate diet, and a low-glycemic-index diet (the glycemic index classifies foods based on how quickly they release sugar, or glucose,
into the bloodstream). They found that people on very low-carb diets
burned the most calories and sustained weight loss—but at a price: The
low-carb diet boosted stress hormones and markers of inflammation,
which could increase the risk of heart disease and other health risks over
the long run.

In my opinion, the Mediterranean diet hits the sweet spot because it's highly palatable, easy to follow, and it emphasizes nutritional attributes that are good for lowering insulin levels and the risk of diabetes and reducing inflammation. The fact is, many of us would happily go to Greece, Italy, Spain, or southern France and spend our hard-earned money on the excellent food there; we wouldn't do this because the food is good for us but because it just plain tastes good! It turns out, it is also good for us, and it offers us the opportunity to love food that loves us back, to get pleasure in the pursuit of health, and health in the pursuit of pleasure. There really is an intersection here where culinary pleasure and good health can converge. That's the sweet spot, and I'd say it's worth parking your fork there.

Once you understand the building blocks of a healthy diet, it will become easier to develop the skills that will help you create one for your plate. For starters, a good maxim to keep in mind: The longer the shelf life of a food product (such as neon-orange cheese puffs), the shorter the shelf life of the person who consumes it regularly. Apart from adhering to that maxim, we should focus on overall nutritional quality, within the full range of food choices that you and other people actually make every day. Without further ado, here are the skills you'll want to develop to create a nutritious dietary pattern that will correct and protect your health-promoting, weight-controlling efforts.

The Skill: Identifying the Fundamentals of Good Nutrition

Just as there are only so many parts to the human body, the same is true of the classes of nutrients the human body needs. Every dietary approach under the sun relies on the same classes of macro- and micronutrients, to one degree or another. Let's discuss the three classes of macronutrients, which are all components of a healthy diet.

Carbohydrate

Carbohydrate is the largest nutrient class, and the greatest source of calories for omnivores and herbivores alike. When omnivores "cut carbs," they tend to cut calories (a lot!), often without realizing it. (When I have closely examined the calorie levels in studies pitting the Atkins Diet against others, the Atkins plan turned out to be the one that restricted calories the most.) But while some people believe that carbohydrates are "bad for you" or promote weight gain, and they avoid them for these reasons, it's a bit like throwing the baby out with the bathwater. It's the quality of the carbs that really matters; after all, carbohydrates include everything from lentils to lollipops.

There are two primary types of carbohydrate: simple carbohydrates (found in table sugar and sugary packaged foods), which your body uses as a quick source of energy that doesn't last long, and complex carbohydrates (found in vegetables, legumes, nuts, and whole grains), which provide a longer-lasting form of energy. Both forms provide much of the energy needed for physical activity and the functioning of your organs. For the most part, though, foods that qualify as sources of complex carbohydrates contain far more nutrients than their simple cousins, making them a healthier, more satisfying choice.

From the *Things-You-Never-Knew-You-Never-Knew* Files

The satiety threshold (i.e., the amount it takes for us to feel satisfied) is higher for sugar than for other food components. As a result, with simple carbohydrates (such as sugary cereals or cookies), it's easy to eat more than you intended to and consume excess calories from these foods.

Complex carbohydrates are high in fiber, which is indigestible and calorie-free, but still takes up considerable space in our stomachs. Soluble fiber (a.k.a. viscous fiber)—abundant in oats, barley, legumes, beans, fruits, and vegetables—is really our best friend, because it slows the entry of sugar and fats into our bloodstream. This enhances feelings of fullness from any given portion (which may prevent overeating) and confers metabolic benefits, including lower blood sugar and blood insulin levels, lower blood lipids/cholesterol, and lower blood pressure. By contrast, insoluble fiber—found in bran, whole grains, nuts, cruciferous vegetables (such as broccoli and cabbage), and the skins of fruits and vegetables—tends to keep things moving efficiently through our digestive system. As you can tell, both are good for you!

Want proof of the power of fiber? Recent research from the European Prospective Investigation into Cancer and Nutrition, which involved 452,717 men and women, found that those with a higher fiber intake had a lower mortality rate, particularly from circulatory, respiratory, and inflammatory diseases, over a twelve-year period. Every 10-gram increase in fiber consumption conferred a 10 percent lower risk of overall mortality. Another branch of the investigation found that people who consumed the highest amounts of fiber had a lower risk of heart disease; in this case, each 10-gram increase in fiber consumption was correlated with a 15 percent lower risk.

Also within the category of complex carbohydrates are whole grains, which tend to be high in fiber and contain healthy oils, health-promoting phytochemicals (plant-based compounds), vitamins, and minerals. Consuming a diet that's rich in whole grains has been linked to a decreased risk of developing cholesterol abnormalities, type 2 diabetes, heart disease, stroke, obesity, and various cancers. It's best to have at least three daily servings of whole grains—options include amaranth, barley, brown rice, cracked wheat, farro, millet, oats, quinoa, spelt, and whole wheat, among others. It's my personal opinion that all of your grain servings should come from whole grains (as opposed to refined grains), with rare exceptions.

The Skinny on Glycemic Measures

In recent years, more and more people have been paying attention to the glycemic effects of food—the extent to which eating a particular food will tend to raise blood sugar levels in the period following the meal. Some people even use the glycemic index (GI) and/or the concept of glycemic load (GL) to guide their dietary choices—which can be good or bad, depending on how they do it. As with a hammer or saw, these tools are only as good as the person's ability to use them.

Foods that are high in refined starches and/or added sugars tend to have a high glycemic effect, which can lead to hormonal swings that trigger repeated cycles of hunger and cravings. Foods that have low glycemic effects—including whole grains, beans, lentils, vegetables, most fruits when eaten whole, lean protein sources, and healthful oils—have the opposite effect, helping to keep blood sugar and related hormones (such as insulin) stable; they also help prevent cravings, while controlling hunger. But here's where it gets tricky: Some foods (such as carrots, apples, chickpeas, walnuts, black beans, and strawberries) have a relatively high GI but a low GL. Avoiding these so-called high-GI foods can lead you down the wrong dietary path, given how healthy and nutritious they are.

Here's how I look at it: The GI is like body weight, and the GL is like body mass index, or BMI. Knowing someone's weight isn't very meaningful unless you also know how tall she is, in which case you can consider the person's weight relative to her height (BMI)— a more meaningful measure. The same thing is true of the GI versus the GL, which adjusts the GI for the amount of food that's being eaten. So while carrots do have a relatively high GI (47), they have a very low GL because you'd have to eat a bushel of carrots to get the blood sugar spike that's suggested by the GI.

It's fine, then, to let the GI guide you to better choices within food categories where nutrition varies widely, such as breads, ce-

(continued)

reals, sauces, and dressings. But overall, GL is a more useful measure because it compares the effects on blood sugar of comparable and realistic amounts of different foods. On the GL scale, most foods widely recognized as nutritious get a predictably low score. If you focus on the overall nutritional quality of foods, and choose wholesome, down-to-earth foods, mostly plants, as much as possible—the GL will tend to take care of itself.

Protein

Of the three classes of macronutrients, protein confers the greatest, and longest-lasting, feeling of fullness, calorie for calorie. This is partly because it takes our bodies longer to digest protein than it does other macronutrients. While there is a limit to how much protein we should eat, placing an appropriate emphasis on high-quality sources (such as fish, lean poultry, lean meats, eggs, low-fat dairy products, legumes, nuts, seeds, and soy foods) can help foster satiety and reduce the calories it takes for us to feel full, which can help with weight control. Most people in the United States consume too much protein. All of us should try to keep protein intake in the optimal zone—0.6 to 1.0 gram per kilogram of body weight in adults daily. (Keep in mind: 1.0 kilogram equals approximately 2.2 pounds.) For the average adult weighing 70 kilograms, or approximately 155 pounds, this would mean roughly 60 grams of protein in a day; about 7 to 8 ounces of any meat or 3 to 4 cups of cooked lentils would provide that much. Other foods provide less concentrated protein, but it all adds up over the course of the day.

Fat

Fat is the last macronutrient. In our culture, it might as well be a four-letter word, considering how maligned it's been, historically speaking. There's no question that consuming too much fat can be harmful to our health and our waistlines; after all, 1 gram of fat contains 9 calories, compared to 4 calories in 1 gram of carbohydrate or protein. But our bodies do need some dietary fat to perform a variety of functions, including making hormones and cell membranes, aiding digestion, promoting the absorption of fat-soluble vitamins, and maintaining skin health. Yet all dietary fat is not created equal. There are healthy fats such as monounsaturated fats (in olive and canola oils) and polyunsaturated fats (from omega-3 fatty acids and vegetable oils). In fact, research from Wageningen University in The Netherlands found that when people at risk for metabolic syndrome followed a diet high in saturated fats for eight weeks, they experienced an increase in expression of genes involved in inflammatory processes; by contrast, those who stuck with a diet rich in monounsaturated fats had greater expression of anti-inflammatory genes, accompanied by a decrease in low-density lipoprotein, or LDL (the "bad" artery-clogging) cholesterol.

Among the healthiest fats on the planet are omega-3 fatty acids—eicosapentaenoic acid (EPA) and docosahexaenoic acid (DHA)—which are present in cold-water fish such as salmon, albacore tuna, mackerel, lake trout, herring, sardines, and anchovies. Walnuts, flaxseeds, tofu, and canola oil contain another type of omega-3 fatty acid called alpha-linolenic acid. Consuming omega-3s may reduce the risk of heart disease and inflammation throughout the body, and they're beneficial for cognitive function and mood as well. Unfortunately, our intake of omega-3 fatty acids, which are highly perishable, is on the decline. Meanwhile, consumption of saturated fats and omega-6 fatty acids, which have a long shelf life and are abundant in processed foods, has been on the rise in modern times; these fat sources can promote harmful inflammation. Research suggests that a healthy balance occurs when the ratio of omega-6 fatty acids to omega-3 fatty acids in the diet is between 1:1 and 4:1; the trouble is that the average American's dietary pattern has a ratio of about 17:1.

By contrast, saturated fats (in meat and full-fat dairy products) and trans fats (in many commercial baked goods, snack foods, and fried foods) have long been known to raise levels of unhealthy LDL, increasing your risk for heart disease and stroke; they also increase hidden inflammation throughout the body, which raises the risk of many forms of cancer. That's why it's important to restrict your intake of saturated fats and to eliminate trans fats from your diet as much as possible. When it comes to your total fat intake, an even split between monounsaturated fats and polyunsaturated fats is a reasonable target.

Healthy Eating by the Numbers: A Summary

- Less than 30 percent of the day's total calories should come from fat (less than 7 percent of daily calories from saturated fat and less than 1 percent from trans fat).
- Forty-five to 60 percent of your daily calories should come from carbohydrates, mostly complex carbohydrates.
- Fiber intake (for adults) should be 25 to 35 grams per day.
- At least half, if not nearly all, your daily grain consumption should come from whole grains.
- Aim for five to eight servings of fruits and vegetables per day, ideally different-colored ones so you can get your fair share of phytochemicals.
- Fifteen to 30 percent of your daily calories should come from protein.
- Have at least two servings of dairy products per day, preferably fat-free or low-fat versions.
- Drink approximately 64 ounces of water per day.
- Sugar intake (added sugars, that is) should be less than 10 percent of your total calories.
- Try to keep your salt intake under 2,400 milligrams per day.
- If you do drink, consume alcohol in moderation: one drink per day for women, up to two per day for men (Note: One drink is defined as a 12-ounce serving of beer, a 5-ounce glass of wine, or 1.5 ounces of liquor.)
- Eat three to four servings of beans and legumes per week.
- Have fish and shellfish three to four times per week.
- Limit your meat (beef, pork, lamb) intake to no more than two meals per week.
- Eat a serving of nuts and seeds four to five times per week.

The Skill: Reshaping Your Plate

We're living in the midst of an obesity epidemic, with ever-present threats to our waistlines. So it's vital that we pay attention to what's on our plates. A prudent, easy-to-remember approach is to fill three-quarters of your plate (at lunch or dinner) with vegetables, salad, and whole grains (in equal proportions, or with more vegetables and salad than whole grains), and reserve the last quarter for a lean protein (nothing larger than the size of your fist). To help us determine the proper ratio of foods in our diet, in 2011 the U.S. Department of Agriculture replaced the food guide pyramid with the "My Plate" concept (www.choosemyplate.gov). While it doesn't spell out precise serving sizes, it does show a healthy proportion of foods from different categories. This guidance is sorely needed, especially since only 1.5 percent—yes, 1.5 percent!—of Americans are getting the recommended daily intake of both vegetables and fruits.

There's nothing wrong with having repetition in your meals. It can simplify your life by taking the guesswork out of deciding what to eat. As long as it's a healthy pattern and it continues to satisfy you, feel free to stick with the meals that work for you. To improve the quality of each meal, you can use these guidelines for a healthy division of portions. Choose from the following categories of foods and fill your plate accordingly:

Vegetables (half your plate)

Choose leafy greens (such as green lettuces, spinach, kale, and collard or turnip greens), artichoke, zucchini, squash, carrots, onions, bell peppers, mushrooms, eggplant, and cruciferous veggies (such as broccoli, cauliflower, cabbage, and Brussels sprouts).

Whole grains or starchy vegetables (a quarter of your plate)

Choose brown rice, quinoa, barley, whole wheat bread, whole-grain pasta, or couscous; or peas, corn, potatoes (sweet or russet), turnips, rutabaga, or parsnips.

Lean protein (a quarter of your plate)

Choose one serving (approximately 3 ounces) of cooked fish, seafood, chicken or turkey breast (no skin), pork loin, lean beef, tofu, soybeans, eggs, lentils, black beans, kidney beans, almonds, cottage cheese, or yogurt.

You'll notice that fruit is missing from the picture. It's an excellent choice for dessert—it's sweet, filling (thanks to its high water content), and very nutritious. So consider having a bowl of fresh berries for dessert or a baked apple or broiled grapefruit—and call it a meal!

The Calorie Equation

For the record, yes, calories do count. They really do. While prominent voices such as Timothy Ferris and Gary Taubes seem inclined to debate the nature of the calorie, I don't see it that way. This is fundamentally about the laws of physics, the laws of the universe: A calorie is, incontrovertibly, now and forever, a calorie, and "calories in versus calories out" does matter in the weight-management picture. Remember the Twinkie diet that grabbed headlines in 2010? In an experiment on himself, a professor of human nutrition at Kansas State University lost 27 pounds in ten weeks by subsisting almost exclusively on Twinkies and other "junk" food. The critical aspect of his plan: He consumed fewer calories than he burned, so he lost weight. This certainly isn't a healthy way to do it, but it proves that ultimately calories do matter.

That being said, the quality of calories matters in addition to the quantity, because nutrition matters to health. The quality also tends to influence the quantity we consume, because wholesome foods help us fill up on fewer calories. When we talk about food, the scientific measure we use is the kilocalorie—Europeans use the term *kilojoule*—that is, the amount of energy that's required to raise the temperature of 1 kilogram of water 1 degree Celsius at sea level. This is the reality: When more energy is taken into the body (from food) than is used by all energy-expending processes (including basic body functions and physical activity), the surplus is converted into body fat. But here's where people get confused: Two people who have the same calorie intake and exercise habits can experience different results; one may gain weight, while the other won't, and people will say, "See, calorie balance doesn't really matter!" But the weight-related results stem from the efficiency of each person's metabolism—the body's internal calorie-burning machine—so the amount of calories that are enough for you to maintain your weight may be different from that of your neighbor who is the same height and weight.

So debating whether a calorie is a calorie, depending on the source of food it comes from, is the wrong question. A better question is: What types of foods will enhance my energy and well-being today while promoting better health for tomorrow? (The answer: It's not Twinkies!) Another good question is: How can I fill up on healthy, satisfying foods that will fight diseases and help me feel better, for a reasonable number of calories? Keep reading, and you'll discover the answers.

From the *Things-You-Never-Knew-You-Never-Knew* Files

Studies show that foods we eat at one time can influence the glycemic effects of foods that we eat at another time. Given that consuming soluble fiber blunts your blood sugar response, if you eat an oat cereal (that's rich in soluble fiber) for breakfast, your body will have a lower glycemic response to whatever you eat for lunch. That's probably something you didn't know—and it's a win-win proposition, any way you look at it.

The Skill: Exercising Portion Control

Now you know that keeping your body weight in the optimal range, which is vital for good overall health, involves achieving the proper balance between calories in (those you consume from food) and calories out (those you expend through physical activity). This, of course, means it's important to control calories on both sides of the energy balance equation. But in the modern age, it's very easy to eat more calories than you expend (even through intense exercise). So portion control (and hence, calorie control) is nonnegotiable. You may not even be aware of just how much portion sizes of prepared foods and restaurant meals have increased over the decades. We're living in an age where our food supply has become "super-sized," in part because we like to feel as though we're getting our money's worth. As a result, we're faced with muffins and bagels that are the size of doorstops, hamburgers that resemble a child's baseball mitt, and soft drink servings that are the size of small watering cans. Given these developments, it's not surprising that many people are consuming lots of extra calories from everyday foods—often without realizing it.

This effect has been reproduced numerous times in the lab. For example, in a study involving thirty-two adults, researchers at Pennsylvania State University had participants eat their main meals in a controlled setting for two consecutive days over three weeks, while varying the portion sizes of the foods and beverages served by 50 to 100 percent: When they increased portions by 50 percent, the people consumed 16 percent more calories over the course of the day; when they increased the serving size by 100 percent, the participants consumed 26 percent more calories on a given day. The take-home message: We often eat or drink much of what's put in front of us, whether or not we consciously want it. This can become an entrenched habit before you know it. Given these findings and our super-sized way of living, it's time for a refresher course on what a sensible portion size looks like:

Food: Whole grains

Serving size: 1 slice of whole wheat or another whole-grain bread, ½ cup cooked whole grains or pasta, 1 cup whole-grain cereal

Real-life references: 1 whole-grain bagel, biscuit, or muffin = hockey puck; 1 cup cereal or popcorn = baseball; ½ cup whole-grain pasta, rice, or couscous = lightbulb; 1 waffle or pancake = compact disc

Food: Fruit

Serving size: 1 medium piece of fresh fruit; ½ cup canned, cooked, or chopped fruit; ¼ cup (or 1 ounce) dried fruit

Real-life references: 1 medium apple or orange = tennis ball; ½ cup berries or grapes = lightbulb; 1 ounce dried fruit (including raisins) = golf ball

Food: Vegetables

Serving size: 1 cup cooked or raw vegetables; 1 cup salad greens; 1 small baking potato

Real-life references: 1 small potato or sweet potato = computer mouse; 1 cup of cooked or raw vegetables or leafy greens = baseball

Food: Dairy and eggs

Serving size: 1 cup milk or yogurt; 1 ½ ounces hard cheese; ½ cup ricotta or cottage cheese; 1 egg

Real-life references: 1 cup of milk or yogurt = baseball; 1 ½ ounces hard cheese = 3 dice; ½ cup ricotta or cottage cheese or frozen yogurt = lightbulb

Food: Meat, fish, or poultry

Serving size: 3 ounces cooked

Real-life references: 3 ounces cooked steak or chicken = deck of cards; 3 ounces cooked fish = checkbook

Food: Nuts and seeds

Serving size: 1 ounce (¼ cup) nuts and seeds; 2 tablespoons peanut butter or other nut butter

Real-life references: ¼ cup almonds or other nuts = golf ball; 2 tablespoons nut butter = two tips of your thumb

Food: Beans and legumes

Serving size: ½ cup cooked beans, lentils, or peas; 2 tablespoons hummus

Real-life references: ½ cup cooked beans or legumes = lightbulb; 2
tablespoons hummus = golf ball

Foods: Oils and added fats
Serving size: 1 tablespoon butter, margarine, or salad dressing
Real-life references: 1 tablespoon butter, margarine, or salad dress-
ing = poker chip

Now that you know how to shape your plate and what a proper portion size looks like, you have the knowledge necessary to develop the
skills involved in preparing or assembling healthy meals.

A Menu for Putting Your Fork to Good Use

Here are examples of what a healthful meal pattern might look like
over the course of three days:

Breakfast: 1 cup cooked plain oatmeal, topped with 1 tablespoon chopped walnuts, 1 teaspoon brown sugar or cinnamon,
1 cup mixed berries; coffee or tea with fat-free milk

Lunch: Tomato stuffed with tuna salad (made with Dijon mustard and fat-free plain yogurt instead of mayo); 5 whole-grain
crackers

Dinner: Grilled chicken with caramelized onions and sun-dried
tomatoes on whole-wheat pita;* cucumber, tomato, red onion,
and kalamata olive salad; baked apple for dessert

Breakfast: 1 cup whole-grain cereal with ½ cup skim milk; 1
orange or banana; coffee or tea with fat-free milk

Lunch: Spinach salad with lentils, feta, and walnuts*

Dinner: Grilled salmon, cooked quinoa, sautéed zucchini, fresh
garden salad; fresh fruit or fruit salad for dessert

(continued)

Breakfast: 2 eggs cooked over easy; I slice whole-grain toast with a little Smart Balance spread; I cup fresh strawberries; coffee or tea with fat-free milk

Lunch: Dijon chicken salad;* 5 whole-grain pita chips

Dinner: Pesto shrimp and pasta primavera;* tossed garden salad; fresh berries for dessert

*Recipe in chapter 8.

The Skill: Putting Fullness on Your Side

The single best way to control the quantity of food you eat is to improve the *quality* of the food you eat. Foods that pack lots of calories into small spaces, as most processed foods do, make it harder to feel full, and thus make it easy to overeat. In contrast, foods with a low energy density, which distribute their calories across a larger volume, tend to have the opposite, beneficial effect of filling us up with fewer calories.

You should also eat foods with a high "satiety index" (providing feelings of satisfaction and fullness)—look for high-quality proteins, high water content (grapes or other fruits), lots of air (think popcorn or puffed rice cereal), and a low glycemic load (a slow rise in blood glucose levels after eating). We also fill up faster on these foods, which tend to be close to nature and free of artificial flavorings, additives, and significant quantities of added sugar and/or salt. Another good strategy is to begin meals with a leafy green salad and low-calorie dressing or a broth-based soup to help curb your appetite and reduce your calorie intake from the main event (the entree).

The Skill: Thinking About Your Drinks

Study after study has found that people don't naturally compensate for the calories they consume from beverages by consuming less food. As a result, liquid calories are often excess calories, so it's wise to pay attention to the kinds of beverages you consume. That doesn't mean you should always drink only calorie-free beverages, but make a habit of considering what else they have to offer in the way of nutrients or health benefits.

As an adult, most of your fluid intake should come from water, seltzer, and other calorie-free options. Water is the most plentiful substance in the body, accounting for about 60 percent of an adult's body weight, and an essential part of the diet. Our bodies have no way to store water, so we need to constantly replenish the fluids we lose through sweat, breathing, urination, and other bodily functions. This means we should drink at least eight cups of water every day, more when the weather is hot or when we exercise or play sports. If you don't like the taste of plain water, add a wedge of citrus fruit, cucumber slices, or a small splash of 100 percent juice.

Next on the hierarchy of smart beverage choices are tea, coffee, and skim milk. Tea and coffee both offer antioxidants and caffeine (healthy in moderation), while skim milk, almond milk, and soy milk are loaded with calcium. Research suggests that green tea's EGCG (short for epigallocatechin-3-gallate) is a powerful antioxidant that can protect your health; moreover, the caffeine in green tea can raise your metabolism (conferring a 10 to 20 percent boost in your calorie-burning capabilities for up to two hours) and promote fat burning. So green tea is a beverage worth drinking! The next, smaller level of beverages includes 100 percent fruit juices. While fruit juices do contain vitamins, they also tend to be fairly high in calories, and a glass of OJ doesn't have the fiber you'd get from eating a whole orange. On our beverage hierarchy, sodas are in last place because they offer nothing in the way of nutrients but plenty of calories and sugar. Diet soda is slightly better—but remember: Even though it's calorie-free, it has no nutritional value.

Be discriminating about the liquid calories you consume; if a beverage doesn't offer nutritional or health benefits, think twice about drinking it. Trimming the calories you consume from beverages will help you more easily shave off excess weight. In fact, research from the Johns Hopkins Bloomberg School of Public Health, in Baltimore, found that when adults reduced their liquid calorie consumption by just one sugar-sweetened beverage per day, they lost weight over six months, without changing anything else about their diets. That's an easy fix to make.

To Supplement or Not to Supplement, That Is the Question

In recent years, the notion that supplements help—or at least don't hurt—has taken a beating. First came a long line of clinical trials suggesting a lack of benefit and the potential for harm from high doses of select nutrients. Then came studies showing associations between multivitamin use and adverse outcomes—in particular, a higher rate of breast cancer among women. Since we've never had clear and compelling evidence of supplements' benefits, even a hint of potential harm was enough to argue pretty powerfully against the routine use of multivitamins. I stopped taking them and stopped universally recommending them to my patients.

The most plausible reason for their potential to do harm relates to what I think of as "nutritional noise": Imagine that a great electric-guitar player from a rock band, a top-notch sax player from a jazz ensemble, and a virtuoso cellist from a symphony orchestra were to play their own brand of music simultaneously. The result of this musical mish-mash would be unpleasant noise. In putting together multivitamin supplements, manufacturers have chosen the dose, the preparation, and the variety of nutrients and taken them all out of their native context (whole foods). If the nutrients are assembled the wrong way, they might clash, and nutritional noise could be harmful.

Confusing matters, a recent study on supplements grabbed headlines in a positive way: A randomized, blinded, placebo-controlled intervention involving nearly fifteen thousand male physicians in the United States found that daily multivitamin use is associated with an 8 percent reduction in the overall rate of cancer. This was statistically significant, although barely so.

(continued)

My opinion is that the decision about whether to take a multi-vitamin should be made individually, based on a discussion between patients and their doctors. I do recommend multivitamin supplements on a case-by-case basis for my patients—if they have major gaps in their nutrient intakes or very inconsistent eating habits, for example. But, here's the bottom line: while an 8 percent decrease in cancer rate may seem significant, it doesn't come close to the 80 percent reduction in the risk of all chronic diseases that you can get from optimal use of your feet (being active), forks (eating well), and fingers (not smoking). So, in the final analysis, a healthy lifestyle still trumps the use of multivitamin supplements any day of the week.

THE DISEASE-PROOF TO-DO LIST:

- Choose wisely from different classes of macronutrients (complex carbohydrate, lean protein, and healthy fats).
- Create a healthy plate with the proper ratio of foods—half veggies, one-quarter whole grains or a starchy vegetable, one-quarter lean protein.
- Exercise portion control so you don't accidentally overeat.
- Fill up on healthy foods that are naturally low in calories, such as fruits and vegetables.
- Make it a point not to drink your calories—unless the beverage offers substantial nutritional value.

• Five •

Bringing Your Head to the Table

The Challenge: In a modern world where multitasking and consuming highly processed foods run rampant, it requires a dedicated and conscious effort to eat well.

The Right Response: Cultivate an awareness of your food choices and modify your personal environment so that eating well comes naturally.

The Relevant Skills: Identifying the role emotions play in your eating habits; finding ways to fulfill your emotional needs without food; adopting the right mind-set before you eat; modifying your environment so it becomes easy to eat healthfully; practicing the art of conscious eating; and minimizing distractions while eating.

When you consider that food is a source of sustenance, energy, nurturance, pleasure, and so much more, it's amazing how mindless we can be about how we use it. Imagine if you were to find a medication sitting on a counter in your kitchen and you had no idea what was in it or what it could do to you: You probably wouldn't put it in your mouth, right? Somehow, most of us generally don't take the same approach to food.

Granted, we don't need to do this when it comes to real foods such as fruits, vegetables, whole grains, nuts, seeds, legumes, beans, dairy products, and lean sources of protein. But when it comes to packaged foods, we often don't have a clue what's in them—so why eat them without investigating? We tend to be much more particular about things that matter a whole lot less than we are about the construction material for our own bodies and those of our growing children and the fuel that runs every one of our vital functions: food. The relationship each of us has with food is powerful and intimate. If you aren't inclined to share your body with anyone you happen to meet, there's no justification for doing so with food. After all, food literally becomes part of you: Your body builds its own cells out of it. You truly, deeply, and in our culture, yes, a bit madly, are what you eat!

Hopefully, that gives you something new to think about—food for thought, as it were—and that's just the point: putting thinking back into the dietary picture. It makes good sense to think about what foods you put in your mouth, as well as when and how much to eat. It makes good sense to make eating a conscious decision, not just a random occurrence or default activity. To do that, you'll want to become more aware of what's in the foods you choose—and become more attuned to your motivations for eating.

After all, hunger is just one of many possible reasons for eating. Food plays numerous roles in our lives—friend or enemy, reward or punishment, a source of pleasure, pain, comfort, guilt, and more. People tend to eat for reasons that have nothing to do with nourishment, sustenance, or energy. People often eat to relieve boredom or loneliness, to soothe their frazzled nerves or blue moods, or to celebrate. And sometimes people eat for no particular reason whatsoever, except that food is "there."

If you think about not just what to eat but also what's behind your motivation to eat, some reasons deserve to stay on the "worthy" list, while others do not. True hunger, of course, does. But emotional reasons for eating may not. The trouble is, you can't just eliminate an emotional motivation for eating and solve the problem. If you eat to address frustration, for example, and you just take away the food, the frustration is still there. It's important to start developing other sources of pleasure or comfort (or whatever feeling food has been giving you) so you won't *need* to overeat.

To some extent, we're all creatures of habit, and food can become a crutch, a distraction, a pacifier, or a mood-altering substance of choice. At first, it plays this role successfully because the very act of eating can provide a short-term way of calming unpleasant feelings, psychologically and physiologically. It can distract you from what's bothering you as you focus on tasting and experiencing the sensory qualities of what you're eating. Plus, eating foods that you deem to be delicious can literally light up the pleasure centers of your brain, making you feel good (or at least better) but also, in many instances, making you want more. It can also ease the body's stress response. Research at the University of California, San Francisco, found that not only does chronic stress increase the palatability of fatty or sugary comfort food, but consuming comfort food while under stress may calm the body's response to the stress by reducing activity in the hypothalamo-pituitary-adrenal (HPA) axis, which releases stress hormones.

The Skill: Identifying the Role Emotions Play in Your Eating Habits

Keeping a food diary for a week can reveal your eating patterns, but it's especially useful for uncovering emotional factors. Besides recording everything you eat and drink (including the actual quantities) throughout the day, jot down the time, circumstances, what else you were doing, whom you were with, how you felt at the moment you decided to eat, and any other relevant aspects of the experience. This will help reveal your triggers (other than true hunger) for eating, drinking, or nibbling.

As an added incentive, consider this: Research has found that when people consistently self-monitor their eating patterns (by writing down what they eat and drink daily), they're more likely to lose weight, even during high-risk periods such as the holidays. Moreover, researchers at the University of Illinois at Chicago found that overweight women who were the most diligent about keeping a food journal lost more weight than their peers did in a twelve-month weight-loss intervention. Part of this is likely due to the vigilance that results from tracking every morsel and sip that cross your lips. It makes you think twice about whether you're making healthy choices, how intensely you want a particular food or beverage, and how much you really want or need to consume. In other words, it cultivates a more conscious, mindful approach to eating. Keeping a food diary also will help you discover where hidden calories may be lurking in your foods (such as sauces, spreads, dressings, and snacks) and beverages, and it can help you gauge the progress you're making in terms of improving your eating habits over time. (For a sample food diary, see Appendix A.)

Whether you developed an emotional eating habit on your own or learned or observed it growing up—if a family member engaged in stress-related munching or offered you a cookie every time you got upset—it's time to realize that it's an unhealthy and unconstructive habit. It can lead to guilt or shame about overindulging, losing control, or gaining weight. Eating badly can even lead to emotional instability at the level of our neurotransmitters. That's a double (or triple) negative!

If anyone can attest to this, it's a patient named Kim, forty-two, who tends to eat whenever she feels sorry for herself. A hard day is a reason for dessert. Stress at work calls for a candy bar. An argument with her husband is an excuse for French fries. Kim and I have talked about her pattern of emotional eating, and I have reminded her that she is the boss. It's my job to tell her what's what, and the rest is up to her. So I have pointed out that if eating anything under the sun when she's upset ends up making her feel worse, then it doesn't make any sense in the first place! To comfort herself when she's upset, she's doing something that makes her more upset, and that makes her stay upset longer—resulting in a negative ripple effect. Kim has now changed her approach: Whenever she's tempted to engage in emotional eating, she pauses to consider how it will make her feel an hour later. She also fortifies her resolve by having healthy foods handy at all times. By thinking about how her food choices will make her feel after the moment has passed, she has decided that she would rather work through a bout of upset emotions now without having a donut, than feel more upset later about having eaten the donut. It's her epiphany; I just happened to be there when she had it.

The Skill: Finding Ways to Fulfill Your Emotional Needs Without Food

Many people know instinctively if they have a tendency to eat for emotional reasons, but others aren't aware of what's driving them to eat. If you use your food diary to connect the dots—by identifying emotional triggers for eating and pinpointing what you're truly feeling—you can begin to address your underlying emotional needs directly, rather than automatically reaching for food. If you're relying excessively on food for pleasure, ask yourself: What else would bring me pleasure? What other sources of delight or gratification could I incorporate into my life so that I depend less on food for that job? The challenge then is to find healthier ways to fulfill those needs or nurture yourself when you're feeling out of sorts.

If you're stressed out, for example, it's better to try to tackle it head-on with a three-pronged approach. First, stop yourself from imagining worst-case scenarios, since this will simply magnify your stress. Correct negative, irrational thinking—"I messed up that project. Now I'll never get promoted at work"—by reminding yourself that just because you made mistakes, that doesn't mean they can't be fixed; nor does it mean your potential for career advancement is doomed. Next, swing into problem-solving mode if the stress stems from a situation you can do something about—fixing a botched report at work or clearing up a misunderstanding with a friend, for example. (If you can't do anything to remedy the situation, try to learn from the experience and move on as best you can.) Third, try to ease your physiological arousal by exercising, breathing deeply, visualizing yourself in a peaceful place (such as the mountains or the beach), or performing progressive muscle relaxation (in which you systematically tense then relax various muscle groups from head to toe). It also helps to avoid letting stress build up throughout the day by taking short breaks to clear your mind with fresh air or work out some of your tension through physical activity.

From the *Things-You-Never-Knew-You-Never-Knew* Files

If you eat chocolate chip cookies *after* you've done something to put yourself in a good mood, you're likely to eat fewer of them. Researchers at the University of Sussex in the United Kingdom found that when people were put in a positive or neutral mood—the positive mood courtesy of watching a comedy movie clip—before being offered chocolate chip cookies, those in a positive mood ate up to three fewer cookies than those in the control group. Perhaps being in a good mood was rewarding enough.

If you're depressed or anxious, exercise is one of the most effective ways to boost your mood and relieve anxiety. Research at Duke University Medical Center found that when people with major depressive disorder did regular exercise (either supervised or at home), they experienced similar benefits to those taking an antidepressant after a year. Meanwhile, another study from Duke found that regular exercisers were less likely to experience a relapse of depression. And a 2012 study at the University of Georgia found that when women with generalized anxiety disorder did two weekly sessions of resistance training or aerobic exercise, their worry symptoms dropped by up to 60 percent after six weeks. That's powerful medicine, indeed. (If you have trouble lifting yourself from the grip of depression or anxiety on your own, bring this to the attention of your health care provider.)

If you tend to eat when you're bored, find something else that's appealing to do or try to find ways to make the boredom more pleasant—perhaps by listening to music or a lively talk show. You might also try tackling a monotonous task in a place where food is not available. If you're frequently bored in your spare time, think about how you could add more interesting, stimulating activities to your life: Try a new hobby, volunteer for a charity, join a book or hiking club, or take a course in an interesting subject. You might also post on the fridge door a list of things you really enjoy doing (perhaps organizing a photo album, reading an engrossing book, writing poetry, or doing an art project with your kids). That way, the next time you head for a snack out of sheer boredom, you'll be reminded of other options you enjoy. Many of these activities will also help if you're trying to alleviate loneliness with food. If you feel an immediate urge to eat out of loneliness, get out of your food-filled environment and find a way to be around other people for a while—by walking in the park (in the morning or afternoon) or browsing at a bookstore (evenings). Or call an old friend and catch up over a soothing cup of hot tea.

From the *Things-You-Never-Knew-You-Never-Knew* Files

In the moments when you can't resist eating for emotional reasons, it's best to choose foods that are satisfying and rich in nutrients. These include healthy sources of fiber-filled carbohydrates—such as whole grains, vegetables, fruits, beans, legumes, nuts, and seeds—which have the added benefit of helping to keep on an even keel your levels of insulin, cortisol, and key neurotransmitters, which affect mood. This can help restore a sense of calm.

The Skill: Adopting the Right Mind-Set Before You Eat

Your expectations, attitude, or mind-set can affect how satisfied you feel after a meal or snack—and it's not all in your head. If you expect a given meal to fill you up, it's more likely to do so. (This is true even if what you consume is relatively low in calories.) If you expect to be left hungry or unsatisfied, there's more of a chance that will happen. In a study at Yale University, researchers had forty-six participants consume a 380-calorie milkshake on two separate occasions. On one occasion, the participants were told that it was an "indulgent" shake with 620 calories; on the other, they were told it was a "sensible" shake with 140 calories. Blood levels of the hormone ghrelin, which stimulates hunger, were measured at baseline; during the anticipatory phase, when they were asked to look at and rate the (misleading) label of the shake; and after they'd consumed the shake. Those who anticipated an "indulgent" shake experienced a steeper decline in ghrelin after consuming the shake than those who thought they'd had a "sensible" shake. Unsurprisingly, participants' ratings of satiety were consistent with whether they believed they'd consumed an indulgent or a sensible milkshake.

This phenomenon is similar to the research on forcing yourself to smile, whether or not you feel happy: The act of consciously putting a genuine smile on your face (what's called a Duchenne smile, which involves both your mouth and eyes) can trigger real feelings of happiness in your brain by evoking the sensation (or physiological memory) of feeling good.

You can also consciously evoke positive memories of healthy eating episodes from the past to set yourself up for a repeat performance. If you're not a fan of Brussels sprouts but you conjure up a happy memory of eating them with friends on vacation, you're more likely to enjoy them in the future. Indeed, researchers at the University of Birmingham in the United Kingdom found that when people are encouraged to recall positive memories of consuming vegetables, they're more likely to enjoy those vegetables and take a 70 percent larger portion of them in a subsequent eating episode than people who are encouraged to recall nonfood memories.

The Skill: Modifying Your Environment So It Becomes Easier to Eat Healthfully

If you have a tendency to gravitate to the "see-food" diet and eat simply because food is present, keeping food out of sight can help keep it out of your mind and out of your mouth. This is an important step in taking a more intentional approach to eating. Stock your fridge and pantry with only healthy choices. If you must keep chips, cookies, and junk food in your home, put these items in the highest cabinet, so they will be out of sight and out of reach. Keep a bag of baby carrots front and center in your fridge, or a bowl of clementines or apples on your kitchen table or even your desk. This is a way of making the see-food diet work for you by putting nutritious, lower-calorie choices within easy reach.

If you have the skills to identify better food, buy and prepare better food, and train your taste buds to prefer healthier foods, then you will be *mindful* about food before it's ever time to eat. The mindfulness is built into your food selection itself, taking the burden off you. Well-chosen food will help you fill up on fewer calories and keep your mood stable, so there is less incentive for emotional eating in the first place. Think of it this way: Thousands of years ago, our ancestors had emotions, and they may have wanted to eat for emotional reasons. But they had a very different food environment, one that didn't promote excess weight gain or health problems. We can refashion our own personal food environments—through the application of skillpower—so that eating well just happens and doesn't require constant mindfulness or vigilance.

Bring nutritious snacks to work—fresh fruit, nuts, dried fruit, brown rice cakes spread with almond butter, low-fat yogurt and berries, snap peas, hummus—in an insulated bag, to help you resist the temptation of vending machines, coworkers' candy jars, and nearby fast-food restaurants or convenience stores. (Yes, dried fruit and nuts can be concentrated sources of calories, but they have a high satiety index—meaning a relatively small portion can help you feel full and stay full—so eating them may actually help you reduce your total calorie intake.) If you know that a specific food triggers overeating for you, don't keep it at home or at your office; when you want to have it, treat yourself to a healthy portion and give the rest away. Taking these steps will remove the need for willpower and turn making healthy eating decisions into a no-brainer, because your environment will set you up for them. You can get used to those choices and come to prefer them. And little by little, you can get used to looking right past unhealthy foods that others introduce into your day.

The Skill: Practicing the Art of Conscious Eating

It's important to look for mindless patterns of eating in your life (hand-to-mouth engagement that occurs with very little awareness) and put an end to them. Ask yourself: Do you regularly dip into a candy dish on someone's desk at work? Do you often finish food that's left on your child's plate? How many other unnoticed actions are adding to your daily caloric intake? If you're like most people, the answers are probably yes, yes, and plenty. If you've had a habit of eating on automatic pilot, one of the keys to changing this is to do something different, to establish a new pattern that will take over for your previous habit. This might include making a point of putting your hands in your pockets when you walk by the candy dish at work or immediately wrapping up or tossing your child's leftovers before you have a chance to pick at them.

To break the cycle, it also helps to alter your environment. If you often munch at your desk when you're feeling tense or overwhelmed, put something else within reach that helps you relax—whether it's photos of your loved ones, music you enjoy, a stress ball to manipulate, or one of your favorite scents (in the form of a fragrant candle or lotion, for example). When you engage in the same comforting habit day after day or night after night—whether it's snacking on chips at your desk or vegging out with a bowl of ice cream in front of the TV after dinner—you end up rewarding yourself with a substantial dose of the mood-boosting neurotransmitter (brain chemical) dopamine. This pleasurable release of dopamine sets the foundation for continuing this behavior-reward cycle. Your brain encourages you to repeat the behavior so that its pleasure centers can light up like Times Square on New Year's Eve again and again.

To break an entrenched behavior-reward cycle, you need to change your routine. If you often grab a cookie, burger, or milkshake on your way home after a stressful day at work, you could instead play a special CD that helps you decompress. In fact, research at Stanford University found that listening to music strongly "modulates activity in a network of mesolimbic structures involved in reward processing" in the brain, structures that are involved in dopamine release. Or you could take a different route home and stop at a farm stand to pick up some fresh flowers or produce. If you're genuinely hungry after work, pack a healthy snack to enjoy on the trip home. If you're not, you could simply look forward to taking your dog for a walk or going on a leisurely bike ride with friends or family members to help you blow off steam. To become more attentive at the table, serve a meal from the stove or a side table, put the food on the plates, and then carry them to the table. This way, you can avoid the perils of proximity—reaching for more simply because you can. To serve yourself another helping, you'll have to get up from the table, which may make you think twice about how badly you really want to have more. During the meal, eat slowly, chew your food thoroughly, and pause periodically. It helps to put your fork down between bites and pay attention to your body's signals of satiety (a.k.a., feelings of fullness). Rather than aiming to feel truly full after a meal, a better approach is to adopt a concept embraced by the Okinawan culture—which is considerably leaner than ours—the concept of *hara hachi bu*: ending an eating occasion when you're about 80 percent full.

Moreover, research at the University of Washington has found that doing yoga can help with weight control. It's not because of the calories that are burned during the mind-body practice. It's because yoga cultivates mindfulness, including a nonjudgmental awareness of the physiological sensations and psychological motivations that are linked with eating. In short, the state of mind that comes from regularly practicing yoga can help you eat when you're truly hungry, stop when you've had enough, and increase your tolerance for mild hunger without feeling a desperate need to squelch it.

The Skill: Minimizing Distractions While Eating

Generally, the more distractions there are during a meal, the more food you're likely to eat, because you won't be paying attention to how much you're putting in your mouth or whether your internal cues of satiety are registering that you've had enough. In addition, a variety of subtle environmental factors, including the lighting and noise level, can practically conspire to make you overindulge. As my colleague Brian Wansink, PhD, of Cornell University and author of *Mindless Eating*, puts it, "Most of us are blissfully unaware of what influences how much we eat. . . . We all think we're too smart to be tricked by packages, lighting, or plates. . . . That is what makes mindless eating so dangerous. We are almost never aware that it is happening to us."

For example, research suggests that bright light, which is abundant in fast-food joints, has a stimulating effect, which can make you eat faster and consume more calories than you normally would. Meanwhile, some studies indicate that people eat more when music is playing than when there is silence or just conversation. In particular, there's some suggestion that loud, fast music tends to increase consumption of food and drinks because the quick tempo makes people eat faster and ultimately consume more food.

When it comes to watching television, the problem isn't entirely what you may think it is. Sure, watching television gets a bad rap because it's a sedentary activity and it often takes the place of more active pursuits, which is why it's believed to be a major contributor to the obesity epidemic. But the effects on weight—and eating behavior, in particular—go far beyond just sitting still. Watching TV can make you want to snack, thanks, in part, to all those commercials for junk food, soda, and other unhealthy food products (a great example of the power of suggestion). The problem is, when you're munching mindlessly in front of the screen, it's easy to lose sight of how much you're eating because, again, you aren't paying attention to your body's natural signals that you've had enough.

The solution is fairly simple: Don't watch TV while eating a meal. If you want to snack while you're watching TV, have a reasonable serving of a healthy food such as apple slices, crudités, or whole-grain chips, then call it quits. If you feel the urge to continue chewing while watching a program, have sugarless gum. Or keep your hands busy by doing needlepoint, folding laundry, or doing another hands-on activity while you watch.

The steps to bringing your head to the table are simple, and they overlap substantially with the skills and strategies you'll read about in other chapters. Collectively, these skills will help you put your fork to better use for the sake of your health and longevity. You'll be able to gain greater enjoyment from the foods you eat, find new ways to fulfill your emotional needs on a deeper level, and make better, more conscious choices of the foods you choose to chew—resulting in a positive synergistic effect.

THE DISEASE-PROOF TO-DO LIST:

- Figure out how to satisfy your emotional needs without food by doing something else that soothes or excites you.
- Get in the right frame of mind before you eat and expect to be satisfied by a reasonable amount of food.
- Alter your environment—by stocking it with healthy foods—so it's easier for you to eat healthfully naturally.
- Cultivate the art of eating more consciously; fully experience and enjoy your food.
- Minimize distractions while you're eating so you can concentrate on enjoying your meal.

• Six •

Taste Bud Rehab

The Challenge: Our modern food supply influences the foods we want, which means our taste buds grow accustomed to and crave foods that aren't healthy for us.

The Right Response: Reeducate and rehabilitate your taste preferences so you'll want to eat foods that are good for you.

The Relevant Skills: Eliminating stealth sources of sugar and salt from your diet; broadening your taste buds' horizons; managing your cravings instead of letting them manage you; and paying attention to sensory-specific satiety.

When it comes to what you put on your plate, the adage that "familiarity breeds contempt" just doesn't apply. On the contrary, familiarity is a potent determinant of dietary preferences and a powerful reinforcing agent. We tend to like what we know. This is evident at the cultural level: Babies in Mexico grow up learning to like spicy food, while Inuit babies develop a taste for seal. Genetically, we are all more alike than different, but culture can change what we find familiar, and hence what we like. Unfortunately, many of the foods that are abundant in our modern American food supply aren't the healthiest choices. While some people think it's their sweet tooth that gets them into trouble, the real problem is that we have too much sugar, salt, and fat in the modern diet, often where it doesn't belong—we've created a food supply that's over-flowing with ingredients that used to be hard to get.

Once upon a time, food cravings actually meant something. The only sweet foods our Paleolithic ancestors had access to were breast milk (sweetened with lactose) for the first year of life, and fruits and honey after that. All were excellent sources of quick, high-quality fuel, and if craving them helped ensure that newborns found breast milk and every-one else found fruit or fought bees for their honey, it was all for the greater good.

The same principles applied to salt and fat. It was hard to find ex-cess salt in a diet that came directly from nature. Most foods that come directly from nature are rich in potassium and relatively low in sodium, so cravings for salt made sense back then. These days, however, most people in the United States consume too much salt—an average of 3,300 milligrams per day, not including salt that's added at the table, accord-ing to the CDC. To put this in perspective, the recommended limit is between 1,500 and 2,400 milligrams per day, depending on the popula-tion. Much of it comes from foods you might not suspect—breads and rolls, breakfast cereals, pizza, fresh and processed poultry, soups, and the like.

Let's compare modern beef and antelope, which is the meat that's closest to what our ancestors ate. While as much as 35 percent of the calories from beef may come from fat, only about 7 percent of the calo-ries from antelope do. In the Stone Age, fat was a valuable source of fuel, but not so easy to find—so again, craving it was good back then. Further, craving a variety of foods helped ensure our forebears met all their bod-ies' nutrient requirements.

Fast-forward to the modern age—the picture has changed entirely. Since we are all the descendants of people who craved sweet, salty, and fatty flavors for survival, it makes sense that we still have the tendency to crave those flavors today. At the same time, our collective desire for those taste sensations has run amok, thanks to the modern food supply. If we bathe our taste buds in sugar and salt all day long, they become desensitized. As a result, our taste buds need more and more of these flavors just to register the slightest sweet or salty sensation.

To make matters worse, companies in the food industry often work with focus groups and sometimes use brain scans to help determine how to engineer their foods, all in the name of making it difficult for people to stop eating them. So when Frito-Lay told us, "Betcha can't eat just one!" in its commercials for Lay's potato chips, you probably didn't realize the company was placing a pretty safe bet. As my friend, colleague, and former Food and Drug Administration commissioner Dr. David Kessler writes in *The End of Overeating*, "To identify a desirable mix of attributes, the industry assembles taste panels that allow consumers and professionals to dissect a given product's pleasing qualities. The industry calls this 'fingerprinting,' and the technique is used to figure out what proportion of which elements will be acceptable to a consumer."

In a 2005 exposé, reporters from the *Chicago Tribune* investigated the lure of junk food and the lengths to which food manufacturers will go to capitalize on it. In particular, the reporters investigated the enduring appeal of the Oreo, the world's best-selling cookie, which happens to be made by Kraft. While spokespeople for Kraft insisted the company "does not conduct research 'aimed at creating consumer dependency upon any of our products,'" the *Tribune*'s examination of tobacco lawsuit documents found that "[i]n fact, Kraft Foods Inc. and Philip Morris USA have pooled expertise in search of making more-alluring foods and cigarettes since the dawn of their corporate pairing two decades ago." All potential conspiracies aside, the point is: Researchers and manufacturers alike are acutely aware of how the optimal combination of sugar, fat, salt, and other food chemicals can get us hooked on junk foods.

Considering that some people naturally prefer sweeter foods while others prefer saltier items, manufacturers typically try to hit "the sweet spot," so to speak, in terms of tastes, textures, and mouthfeel, so that their product will have the broadest appeal to the greatest number of consumers. As Dr. Kessler notes, "Rewarding foods tend to be reinforcing, meaning that they keep us coming back for more." Manufacturers of processed foods are counting on this. Their goal is nothing short of wanting to profit from our inability to control ourselves when their irresistible food product is in our hands. This is a reality that presents a hidden challenge to eating well in the modern world.

In recent years, evidence has been mounting to suggest that in those who are susceptible, some foods may in fact hijack the brain's reward system in a way that's similar to cocaine, heroin, or other abused drugs. Studies using functional magnetic resonance imaging (fMRI) and positron emission tomography (PET) scans have shown that when people with food addictions either are shown pictures of or eat sweet, salty, or fatty food, the pleasure centers of their brains light up like pinball machines and they stay lit up much longer than in people who don't have a food addiction. This heightened brain activation triggers an intense desire for more of the coveted food.

The Facts on Flavor Preferences

For better or worse, the way we eat is shaped largely by various social influences throughout our lives. From the time we were mere fetuses in our mothers' wombs, we began to develop a taste for certain foods our mothers ate, as the flavors passed to us via the umbilical cord. After we entered the world, breast milk may have transmitted flavors from our mothers' diets, also influencing our budding sense of taste. From early childhood on, our parents and caregivers played a significant role in how our dietary preferences developed, by exposing us to new foods, withholding others, and modeling eating habits. If our parents had less-than-stellar eating habits, there's a good chance we followed their lead with our forks in hand. Then, during the teen years, as we increasingly ventured out into the world with friends, peer influences came into play as well.

Judging by the flavors emphasized in processed foods, you might think there are only two basic taste qualities, but there are in fact five—

sweet, sour, salty, bitter, and umami (or "savory"). Many of us don't naturally choose enough from categories other than sweet and salty. Which
means we may be cheating ourselves, nutritionally speaking, since many
of the healthiest foods on the planet have a naturally bitter flavor (kale,
spinach, eggplant), sour flavor (grapefruit, kiwi, plain yogurt), or an
umami flavor (fish, mushrooms, tofu, green tea).

To some extent, taste preferences are hardwired. While a friend
might like broccoli rabe, you may think it's too bitter—the two of you
have different genes and different taste receptors that may make you
more or less sensitive to bitter tastes. In fact, some people inherit genes
that make their taste receptors intensely sensitive to bitterness, which
may make them less likely to consume bitter foods. For good reason,
these folks are often referred to as "supertasters," because they experience the sense of taste—especially bitter, spicy, or umami flavors—with
greater intensity than most people do. But genetic factors don't tell the
whole story. Individual taste preferences are also influenced by environmental, social, and emotional factors. In a study involving 663 female
twins at the University of Helsinki in Finland, approximately half the
preference for sweet tastes was explained by genetic factors, the rest by
environmental influences that were unique to each twin.

In general, people naturally tend to prefer sweet, salty, and umami
foods and to reject bitter and sour tastes, but these innate penchants can
be changed by experience over time, as you'll see. The trouble in our
culture is that people often associate sweets with comfort or pleasure,
and as we now know, sweet tastes naturally stimulate your appetite. The
same thing can happen with salty foods. (By contrast, bitter and astringent tastes tend to suppress appetite.) Much of this exposure to sugar and
salt is wholly unnecessary: Why, for example, should we eat pasta sauces
or salad dressings that are more concentrated in added sugar than ice-
cream toppings? Or breakfast cereals that are more concentrated sources
of added sodium than potato chips or pretzels? There's no good reason
for this, but it is our reality, and it can cause us to lose our sensitivity to
sugar and salt, respectively.

The Skill: Eliminating Stealth Sources
of Sugar and Salt from Your Diet

Of course, we *do* still need sodium, fat, and a bit of sweetness in our diets, but their abundance in processed foods means the problem for most of us is avoiding too much. The good news is you can sidestep the excess and restore your taste buds to their former state of virtue. By dialing down your exposure to processed foods, you can reverse-engineer the corruption process, rehabilitate your taste buds, and come to love food that's far more likely to do your body good. Your taste buds will adjust to lower thresholds of these flavors, feeling satisfied with lower amounts of salt, sugar, and fat. Over time, the sweet and salty foods you used to eat by the handful may taste *too* sweet or salty to you.

Research suggests that when people stick to a lower-sodium diet for a period of time, they actually develop a preference for less salty foods. Meanwhile, reports from the Iowa Women's Health Study, which has been ongoing since the mid-1980s, showed that women who made the transition to a plant-based, lower-fat diet actually acquired, over a span of months, aversions to many of the processed and fast foods they liked at the start of the study. When changes like these occur, you know you've begun to rehabilitate your taste buds.

Chances are you've experienced this effect yourself or seen it in your family. When people make the transition from whole milk (a hefty source of saturated fat) to skim milk (a far healthier choice), at first they usually find that skim tastes a bit like dishwater (at worst) or watered-down milk (at best). But if they stick with the skim variety for two weeks, their palate usually adjusts; if they stay with it for longer and then taste whole milk, it suddenly tastes too rich and thick to them. In more than twenty years of clinical practice, I have been through this transition with many patients, both adults and children, and the results are impressively consistent. The same thing is true with making small, gradual changes toward more healthful foods in general. Switching to whole grains is easier, for example, when you gradually replace processed grains with whole grains. So the next time you make rice, try blending one-third brown rice and two-thirds white rice; over time, you can gradually adjust the ratio (at a rate you're comfortable with) until you are eating 100 percent brown rice.

You can also cut down on your sugar intake by making your own pasta sauce or salad dressing or choosing healthier ones that contain less of the sweet stuff. Keep in mind that sugar and sodium hide in the unlikeliest of foods. If you learn how to read food labels effectively (see chapter 7), you'll be able to find the sugar and salt you expect as well as that you don't. After all, sugar goes by many different names on food labels—sucrose, fructose, corn syrup, evaporated cane juice, and others. (Keep in mind: Agave syrup, often viewed as having a health halo, is a highly concentrated source of fructose and carries little, if any, health benefits.) Besides looking at the total sugar content on the Nutrition Facts panel, you'll want to examine the ingredients list to see how prominently sugar (or any variations of it) is featured; the higher it is on the list, the more the food product contains. Avoid packaged foods with a Daily Value (DV) of sodium above 5 percent. You can also skip the step of adding salt to a pot of boiling water before cooking pasta; you really don't need it if you simply stir the pasta to prevent it from sticking together.

If you shift steadily to more wholesome foods, you'll reduce the amount of time your taste buds spend immersed in sugar, salt, and food chemicals each day. This change in exposure will almost certainly lead to greater taste sensitivity, which means your taste buds will eventually become satisfied with and come to prefer less sugar and less salt. Before long, you will likely prefer less sweet desserts, too.

The Skill: Broadening Your Taste Buds' Horizons

No matter which tastes you naturally gravitate toward, it is possible to broaden your penchant for certain flavors, especially as you get older.

That's because your taste buds typically become less sensitive as the decades pass, which allows you to enjoy foods that once tasted too strong, bitter, or astringent to you—things such as Brussels sprouts, collard greens, olives, cabbage, turnips, coffee, beer, and the like. Different foods offer different nutrients (and in varying amounts), so you're more likely to meet your body's needs when you consume a more varied diet. With an open mind and the right experiences, you might even come to crave parsnips or rutabagas sautéed in a small amount of low-sodium soy sauce (instead of French fries), a Portobello mushroom burger (instead of a beef burger), or a cinnamon-infused poached pear for dessert (instead of ice cream).

It helps if you try to give yourself reasons to like foods with flavors you don't fully appreciate. For example, if you learn about why kale is good for you (because it's loaded with fiber; vitamins A, C, and K; calcium; iron; and health-promoting phytochemicals, for example), you'll give yourself more incentive to try it and like it. It also helps if you pair foods you really like with ones you don't quite appreciate. So if you're agnostic about beets (or actually dislike them) but you do like blue cheese and walnuts, you might try having them all together, in a spinach salad. Similarly, if you don't like tofu but you love salads or stir-fries, you could try tossing some crumbled tofu into your favorite of either. Some researchers call this "flavor-flavor learning," and it really does work: This conditioning strategy has helped kids learn to like and accept a variety of vegetables, but it works with adults, too.

You can also take the bite out of bitter or sour foods by adding a sprinkle of citrus zest, lemon or lime juice, flavored vinegar, garlic, herbs (such as thyme, fennel, oregano, and rosemary), or spices (ginger, curry powder, paprika, nutmeg). Try roasting Brussels sprouts with a spritz of olive oil and a sprinkling of fine herbs, or serving sautéed kale with a dash of balsamic vinegar. If you don't like eggplant, try adding it into a stew with garbanzo beans, diced roasted tomatoes, and cumin. Don't care for plain yogurt? Try mixing nonfat Greek yogurt with fresh blueberries and a dash of vanilla extract. Whether you serve certain foods cooked versus raw, or roasted versus steamed, can also have a dramatic effect on their flavor. If you don't like steamed broccoli or cauliflower, try having it raw with a tangy mustard sauce or roast it with a splash of olive oil and rosemary, then enjoy its caramelized flavor. Certain cooking techniques (broiling, grilling, and roasting, in particular) can often bring out the natural sugars in bitter vegetables.

The reality is that cultivating a taste for certain foods may require repeated exposure, so be patient. Research at the Monell Chemical Senses Center, in Philadelphia, found that when people consumed a bittersweet beverage once each day for a week, they ended up liking the drink 68 percent more than they did initially. So persistence really does pay off! Once you've tried them several times, unfamiliar foods become familiar, and they can gradually be incorporated into your diet rather seamlessly.

From the *Things-You-Never-Knew-You-Never-Knew* Files

It can take children as many as ten to fifteen tries before they will accept a new flavor—a phenomenon known as "food neophobia"—but the timeline is usually considerably shorter for adults.

The Skill: Managing Your Cravings Instead of Letting Them Manage You

There are two prevailing schools of thought about cravings. The first is that you should give in to them, because they're telling you something about what your body needs. The second is that you should resist them, because they're entirely psychological. Personally, I think both these theories are partially correct, with the caveat that our modern cravings don't mean what they once may have. Meanwhile, cravings can also be psychological, especially when they're about getting pleasure, comfort, or gratification from food instead of from something else. That has nothing to do with what your body needs and everything to do with what your mind and mood need. The real problem, as I see it, is that indulging our cravings too often, whether it's a yen for sweets or a desire for salty foods, can lead us toward foods that divert us from the route to better health and weight control. In the worst-case scenario, it could send our health-promoting efforts on a dramatic detour entirely.

One of my patients, named Helen, calls herself a food addict. Whether or not this is true, Helen certainly has powerful cravings, most often for sweets but sometimes for starchy or salty foods. Helen's cravings tend to occur when she is upset or frustrated or having a bad day; that's when her comfort foods start calling her name. Her cravings also can be triggered by her environment: If Helen goes into a candy store with a friend, for example, even if she has no intention of buying or eating anything, the candy's agenda takes over.

Helen has told me many times about finding herself in situations that just "took control," rendered her helpless, and caused her to eat things she hadn't planned to eat. Without fail, these occurrences end the same way—with feelings of guilt and regret that persist for hours. The irony is that the whole point of giving in to a craving is to get pleasure and satisfaction. But if the net result is *less* overall pleasure, it's a pretty bad strategy. The trouble is, in the exact moment the craving occurs, it's difficult to keep the future, even later that same day, in mind.

The best strategies, then, involve preventing cravings in the first place, finding ways to make them go away when they do occur, and training ourselves to crave foods we truly want to be eating. (Sometimes, managing cravings requires finding other sources of gratification besides food so that your pleasure quotient isn't so dependent on what you chew or sip; for more about this, see chapter 5.) For starters, if you eat regularly—meaning having a healthy, balanced meal or snack every three to four hours—your hunger will be kept in better check around the clock and you'll be less vulnerable to impulse cravings. If cravings do occur, try to wait them out. Many pass in ten to fifteen minutes, so if you can distract yourself in an engrossing activity for that long—whether it's by calling a friend, taking a walk, or playing a game—the yen may disappear entirely before you indulge it. In fact, research from the University of Exeter in the United Kingdom found that a fifteen-minute brisk walk reduced urges for chocolate among regular chocolate eaters. If you must give in to a craving, have a small portion, then wait: Researchers at Cornell University recently found that hedonic hunger (eating for pleasure) is satisfied by a handful of a tasty food, and tends to disappear after fifteen minutes, so long as the memory of indulgence remains.

After having rehabilitated your taste buds, you might find that you can satisfy cravings with less food or better choices. When your sweet tooth starts crying for attention, try eating something naturally high in sugar, such as fruit, or try turning it off by eating a food with a clashing flavor—perhaps half a grapefruit or a sour or bitter orange (like a Seville)—or by switching to a flavor that cleanses the palate (such as a strong mint). If the sweet craving persists, consider indulging mindfully by having a single square of dark chocolate (60 percent cocoa or more) or sorbet instead of ice cream. Similarly, if you crave salt, you might try satisfying the hankering with a cup of miso soup or whole-grain chips instead of the regular variety.

The Skill: Paying Attention to Sensory-Specific Satiety

Having a variety of foods can keep your diet interesting, but having too many choices in a given meal can actually stimulate your appetite and cause you to overeat. This is based on the science of "sensory-specific satiety"— a term you may not have heard before but a concept probably familiar to you. As an example, consider this: How many times have you had room for dessert at the end of a big meal? You might feel too full to eat another bite, but when dessert arrives, suddenly you're looking forward to digging in again. This has nothing to do with having a hollow leg or an extra stomach, but with sensory-specific satiety—the tendency to get full and lose interest in food in a flavor-specific manner but be able to continue eating when flavors and sensory properties of foods (texture, aroma, mouthfeel, and the like) change. In particular, we tend to have extra room for sweets because that's the flavor with the highest threshold for reaching maximum fullness in the first place.

In general, the more foods and flavors you taste, the more you're likely to eat simply to reach the point of satisfaction with each one. That's why it's important to avoid overstimulating your taste buds—and hence your appetite—with too many taste sensations in one meal. Try to limit the number of flavors in a meal to just a few, so that you'll be more likely to feel satisfied and stop eating after consuming a reasonable amount of food. If you enjoy sampling lots of different flavors, it's better to spread them out over consecutive meals or days than over courses in a given meal. The goal is to have variety over time, not variety all at one time. The alternative: an appetite that seems to expand as your belly does.

After all, when you eat multiple flavors at a time, your brain does not say, "Enough! Stop eating!" as quickly as it would if you ate just one or two flavors. The distraction factor that occurs when people shift their attention from one taste to another may also play a role. In an experiment at the University of Liverpool in the United Kingdom, researchers gave thirty-three people a snack of sweet or salted popcorn (their choice). On one occasion they were allowed to eat their popcorn freely; on another, they were interrupted periodically and asked to rate the popcorn they were eating; on two other occasions, their snack was interrupted and they were asked to taste and rate another food with either a similar taste or a different one before resuming their popcorn noshing. Overall, the participants consumed nearly three times more popcorn on the occasions when they tasted other foods, which suggests that the introduction and distraction of sensory variety delayed the "development of satiation," as the researchers put it.

In my clinical practice, I have counseled hundreds of patients who desperately wanted to lose weight. Each time they went on a diet, they shed some weight but eventually gained it back (and sometimes more) when their hunger and cravings went into overdrive. What they didn't know was how to put flavor management on their side to subdue their appetites, and help them fill up on fewer calories. By using flavors strategically and limiting the varieties of tastes you include in any given meal, you can create and consume meals that push your brain and belly's satiety buttons and turn off cravings sooner. Making these changes will help you stick with healthier choices, reform your overstimulated taste buds, and manage your weight more effectively. Those are effects that can appeal to everyone's palate.

THE DISEASE-PROOF TO-DO LIST:

- Eliminate unnecessary sugar and salt from your diet so your taste buds won't crave the stuff as much.
- Expose your taste buds to new, healthy taste sensations by combining new foods and flavors with those you already like.
- Learn to prevent or control cravings by eating healthy meals at regular intervals and distracting yourself or substituting a clashing or palate-cleansing flavor when a craving strikes.
- Limit your taste options in a given meal so you don't overstimulate your appetite.

• Seven •

Shopping for Healthier Foods

The Challenge: Food choices used to be limited to, well, food: edible things that came from nature, things we could recognize and pronounce. Now, faced with a food supply that includes approximately eight hundred thousand foods, including an average of fifty thousand in the typical American supermarket, none of us is savvy and knowledgeable enough to know absolutely everything about the healthy versus the unhealthy.

The Right Response: Learn to find the better choices nestled among the bad ones in every aisle of every supermarket.

The Relevant Skills: Trading up with every class of food; stocking up on healthy staples for your pantry and fridge; learning how to decipher food labels effectively; finding ways to afford good nutrition; and raising nutrition-savvy kids.

It's nearly impossible to assemble or prepare healthy meals at home if you don't have the right ingredients on hand. Eating well really does start with making smart choices at the supermarket, yet many people find grocery shopping challenging for a variety of reasons. My research team at the Yale-Griffin Prevention Research Center has found that people often dread shopping because of the time it takes, organizational challenges, the gap between their current eating habits and their desire to choose healthier foods, or simply a lack of knowledge about how to eat well. Add to these the overwhelming size of many supermarkets, and the challenge is magnified. Then there's the prevailing notion that more nutritious foods cost more, which is sometimes true but often not. Nevertheless, the idea has caught hold, and just believing it dissuades many people from trying to improve their choices. Instead, they continue to buy what they already know.

Unfortunately, the most frequently advertised foods are the most familiar to consumers, and these products generally appeal to adults and kids alike. The tendency to gravitate toward what we know is compounded by the fact that the big food companies pay a premium to put their products in the best locations—right at eye level. As any real estate agent will say: location, location, location! Making matters even more daunting are the many claims on food packaging. Some of them are meaningful; many are not. While the information on food labels can't be outright lies (legally speaking), they can certainly be spun to the positive, blurring the negative or questionable attributes of a particular product to the point where it can be difficult to know what's true and what's not. Too often, many people simply stop trying to make sense of the information.

If anyone can attest to this it's my wife, Catherine, who grew up in southern France, where she learned wonderful Mediterranean French cooking from her mother and aunt. She came to this country when she was fourteen, went on to get her bachelor's degree at the University of California–Berkeley and then her PhD in neuroscience from Princeton University. Yes, I admit it. She's the real brain in the Katz household! Over the course of our twentysomething-year marriage, Catherine has learned just about everything I know about nutrition. We have five children, and since child number three came along, Catherine has devoted the bulk of her time to running our household, including shopping and cooking for the seven of us. That's no easy task, especially given my fussy nutrition standards!

I doubt you'll find a savvier shopper in the whole country, and yet I can remember a time when Catherine would come home from the supermarket with four different loaves of bread and fumes of frustration coming out of her ears. She'd look me in the eye and say, "If you want the most nutritious one of these, *you* figure out which one it is! The first bread has the most fiber but also the most sodium. Is that a good trade-off or a bad one? I can't tell. The second bread has less sodium and pretty good fiber, but it's got high-fructose corn syrup. It's fairly far down the ingredients list, but it's there. The third bread doesn't have added sugar, the fiber is decent, and the sodium isn't bad. But while it says 'zero grams trans fat' on the front of the package, it has partially hydrogenated oil in parentheses on the ingredients list. The fourth bread is a multigrain, but it has the least fiber of all, so I'm not sure any of it is actually whole grain. Which bread is best? Who knows?!"

Seeing that a neuroscientist couldn't pick out a healthy loaf of bread gave birth to an idea I could not let go of: to convene a multidisciplinary panel of top-notch experts in nutrition and public health and have them turn their expertise and the best available science into a nutrition guidance system anyone could use. In 2003, I tried to get the Department of Health and Human Services and other federal agencies to commit to such an enterprise. When the idea didn't gain traction after a couple of years, I turned to Griffin Hospital—a Yale University–affiliated, not-for-profit community hospital, and home to my off-campus lab, the Yale University Prevention Research Center—for financial and administrative support.

Over the next two years, a team of extraordinary scientists came together to empower consumers everywhere to get past food marketing deceptions and be able to identify better nutritional choices at a glance. There were no industry entanglements and no politics involved; with this illustrious group, there was simply a collective passion for creating a system that would serve the public well. Together, we developed an algorithm called the Overall Nutritional Quality Index (ONQI), which scores food products based on their nutrient density. The NuVal Nutritional Scoring System—which has been used to score more than one hundred thousand foods to date—is the public face of this nutrition profiling algorithm, and it's like a GPS for nutrition: It's designed to ensure that anyone who uses it never gets lost or disoriented in the supermarket again. You can find the scores right on the shelf tag below the item, and it won't take long to see that there is an incredible range in nutritional quality in almost every category of food in the supermarket. (Some people will have direct access to NuVal Scores in their local grocery; others may not—but reading about it here equips you with knowledge about how great the range of choices is within specific categories.)

The NuVal System ranks foods on a scale from 1 to 100—the higher the number, the more nutritious the food—across various categories of foods, both packaged foods and fresh items (such as produce and meat). The scoring formula takes into account more than thirty nutrients and nutritional factors, including energy density, fiber content, volume, the quantity and quality of protein, sugar content, fat quantity and quality, vitamins and minerals, and the food's glycemic load. For these and other reasons, a higher score on the NuVal scale indicates a food that is better for you and more likely to help you feel full on fewer calories. Just as you compare prices, you can compare the overall nutritional quality of one product to another within the same category or from diverse categories on the basis of overall nutritional quality.

There are salty snacks (chips, pretzels, cheese puffs, popcorn) that are not very good for you, and salty snacks (made from whole grains, healthful oil, and just a bit of salt) that are much better for you. In this particular category, the scores range from under 10 to around 60—that's a big range. The same is true of crackers, breads, cereals, pasta sauces, salad dressings, yogurts, cookies, and more. As you might expect, salad dressings and pasta sauces earn a fraction of the points that fruits and vegetables do in the NuVal System. And it probably doesn't come as a shock that broccoli, spinach, blueberries, and strawberries all score 100—but so does Yoplait Light Fat-Free (plain) yogurt. It also may surprise you to learn that Post Shredded Wheat Spoon Size, red raspberries, and Dannon Oikos Greek nonfat yogurt (plain) each earns a 91. Perhaps the biggest surprise, however, is the sheer range of scores within a given category of foods, often because of the finer details. For example, regular peanut butter has a higher score than reduced-fat peanut butter because the latter has added sugar and salt. In the bread category, you might expect that Arnold Whole Grain Country White bread would score lower than Pepperidge Farm Farmhouse Soft Oatmeal bread, but the opposite is true: the NuVal Score for the Arnold bread is 39, compared to 18 for the Pepperidge Farm Farmhouse Soft Oatmeal bread, because the Arnold bread contains more fiber, vitamin D, and calcium; less sodium and total calories; and no saturated fat. Another eye-opener: Ragu Old World Style Traditional pasta sauce has a NuVal Score of 51, whereas the company's Light Tomato & Basil pasta sauce has a score of 32. (It gets penalized for added sugar, and the Traditional sauce earns points for containing omega-3 fats.) (For more foods and their scores, check out the Appendix B.)

Besides helping you choose healthier foods, the NuVal System can help you improve your health status in the areas that matter most. In a study published in 2011, researchers from the Harvard School of Public Health tracked the dietary data and health conditions of more than one hundred thousand people from 1986 to 2006. What they found: The people who consistently consumed foods with the highest ONQI scores—the basis for the NuVal System—had a lower risk of chronic disease (including heart disease and diabetes) and of death from any cause over that twenty-year period. Using the system has also enabled many people to lose weight, without changing any other aspect of their lifestyles.

Right now the NuVal System is in approximately 1,700 supermarkets across the country. If you have access to it, you have a shortcut to shopping for healthy foods. If you don't have access to NuVal Scores, you'll have to act as your own nutrition sleuth; read on to learn how. In either case, you'll want to develop the skills that will help you make your time spent shopping as efficient and empowered as possible.

The Skill: Trading Up with Every Class of Food

There is a prevailing view in our culture that if it tastes good, it's bad for you, and that if it's good for you, it tastes bad. This is simply untrue. Some of the best foods and cuisines on the planet are among the most healthful. Dark chocolate alone proves that there are foods to love that love us back! (According to recent research, besides being a rich source of antioxidants, dark chocolate, when consumed in moderate amounts, can improve platelet function and endothelial function, how blood vessels regulate blood flow, and reduce oxidative stress and inflammation, thereby promoting cardiovascular health.) So we need to overcome this bias and get in the habit of choosing foods that foster health while also pleasing our taste buds.

The first step is to improve your choices within every category of foods so that you're selecting tasty, nutrient-rich options that will help you fill up on fewer calories. Indeed, if you want to control the quantity of the food you eat (permanently), the best way to do it without going hungry is to trade up your food quality. The key is to fill up on foods that are naturally low in calories but loaded with nutrients and healthy components (such as water, fiber, and protein).

Fortunately, there are plenty of choices that fit this profile, including fruits and vegetables from every color on the spectrum. The vivid pigment in these brightly hued fruits and veggies indicates a greater presence of health-enhancing nutrients. For example, research from the University of Wisconsin found that orange carrots contain more health-protective beta-carotene than the wild white carrot, a difference that stems from genetic variations in the carrots themselves and the orange variety's inherent pigment. The compounds that give produce its rainbow of colors are called phytochemicals, and they have a wide array of beneficial effects on health, including powerful antioxidant and anti-inflammatory properties. Research suggests that a higher intake of phytochemicals can lower the risk of many chronic diseases including heart disease, diabetes, and certain types of cancer; it can also bolster immune function.

Some specific examples of trading up: It's better to choose sweet potatoes rather than russet potatoes; go for spinach or arugula instead of iceberg lettuce. Lean bacon is better than regular bacon; whole wheat pasta is healthier than white pasta; brown rice is better than white rice (brown rice still has the healthy bran, so it retains more nutrients); and whole-grain tortillas are a more nutritious choice than white flour ones. On the dessert front, dark chocolate is a healthier choice than milk chocolate (because the dark stuff contains a higher concentration of cocoa, less sugar, less "bad" saturated fat, and more beneficial antioxidants).

Across any given category of food, specific items can vary widely in their nutrition and calorie content, so you'll want to pay attention to the details in order to make smart choices. After all, breads can be high in fiber or low in fiber; they can contain lots of added sugars or salt, or not. Just as milk can be high in fat (as with whole milk), have reduced fat (2 percent milk), be low-fat (1 percent), or be fat free (as with skim milk), meats can be high in fat, lean, or extra lean. The white meat of chicken or turkey is generally lower in fat and calories, just as cuts of red meat from the round or loin are; when choosing ground meat, look for "extra lean." When it comes to deli meats, turkey breast and lean ham (low sodium) are healthier choices than salami, bologna, corned beef, or pastrami.

On the fish front, wild salmon, trout, mackerel, sardines, anchovies, and tuna are the best sources of anti-inflammatory omega-3 fatty acids, but all forms of fish and seafood are good sources of lean protein. Although some fish, such as swordfish and tilefish, are high in mercury (which can be harmful to developing brains), the research suggests that the benefits of eating fish outweigh the potential risks from contamination. (Still, if you are pregnant or have young children, consult your doctor about which fish choices are right for you.)

Even pure fats can vary in their health value. If you use heart-healthy olive or canola oil, instead of (artery-clogging) butter or margarine, for cooking, you'll do your heart and the rest of your health a huge favor.

Similarly, you'll want to choose breads, cereals, and crackers made of whole grains. For the record, lean meats, fish and seafood, leafy greens (such as spinach, kale, and Swiss chard), colorful fruits and vegetables, whole grains, and heart-healthy oils all feature prominently in the Mediterranean diet.

The Skill: Stocking Up on Healthy Staples for Your Pantry and Fridge

To expedite wholesome home-cooked meals, you'll want to have the right ingredients available. In addition to the major food groups—whole-grain breads, fruits, vegetables, lean poultry and meat, eggs, low-fat milk, yogurt, and cheeses—you'll want to keep staples such as mustard, hummus, sun-dried tomatoes, horseradish, Parmesan cheese, fat-free plain yogurt, olives, garlic, and fresh herbs in your fridge, and lots of frozen fruits and veggies in your freezer. A well-stocked pantry is also essential: It puts all the items you need for healthful cooking, baking, and snacking within arm's reach. A well-stocked kitchen helps create a safe nutritional haven in your home so that you can quickly pull together healthful meals without succumbing to adverse influences from the outside world.

By having these options at your fingertips 24/7, healthful eating at home becomes the path of least resistance. Simply open your cabinet doors or walk into your pantry, grab the right items, and within twenty minutes you can have a delicious, nutritious meal on the table. It's a new way to look at fast food! With that goal in mind, here's what I recommend for every well-stocked pantry:

- Canola and olive oils
- Whole-wheat couscous and pasta
- Dried lentils and barley
- Dried beans of various types
- Brown rice and wild rice

- Canned garbanzo beans, cannellini beans, black beans, and kidney beans
- Canned whole plum tomatoes, diced tomatoes, and crushed tomatoes
- Tomato paste
- Canned corn and peas
- Canned tuna and salmon (in water)
- Low-fat, low-salt canned soups or stews
- Balsamic vinegar, red wine vinegar, apple cider vinegar
- Unsalted bread crumbs
- Fat-free, low-sodium vegetable broth and chicken broth
- Low-sodium soy sauce
- Flour, cornmeal
- Brown sugar, granulated sugar
- Baking powder and baking soda
- Pure vanilla extract, pure almond extract, pure orange extract
- Unsweetened cocoa, bittersweet chocolate (at least 60 percent cacao), semisweet chocolate chips
- Canned evaporated skim milk and nonfat powdered milk
- Canned pumpkin
- Whole-grain pancake mix
- Oatmeal and steel-cut oats
- A variety of low-fat, whole-grain cereals
- Honey and maple syrup
- All-fruit preserves
- Nut butters
- Almonds, walnuts, soy nuts (roasted soybeans)
- Flaxseeds, sunflower seeds, pumpkin seeds
- Dried fruit such as raisins, apricots, cherries, and figs
- Low-fat, low-sugar granola bars
- Baked fat-free whole-grain pretzels, chips, or crackers
- Salsa
- Brown rice cakes
- Low-fat microwave popcorn

Even with these items, you'll want to do a careful assessment of the ingredients and Nutrition Facts, because as you now know, not all tomato paste or canned corn, for example, is created equal.

To shop efficiently and help avoid making impulse purchases at the store, plan ahead by writing down a menu for the week and then creating a shopping list of ingredients you'll need to prepare the meals you have in mind. You'll save time by doing a big weekly shop, rather than having to go more often if you don't have the right items on hand. If you keep a list on your computer or smartphone of healthy items or brands you buy regularly, you can use it week after week without having to reinvent the wheel. Each week, decide which foods you really need to buy and which you can skip.

If you organize your shopping list according to sections of the grocery store (produce, dairy, breads, meat and fish, and so on), you'll be able to move swiftly and smoothly along. You've probably heard that you should spend the bulk of your time shopping along the perimeter of the grocery store. It's sensible advice, given that this is where the most wholesome choices reside—fruits and vegetables, seafood, poultry, dairy products, and eggs. But that doesn't mean you should avoid the middle aisles entirely. In fact, if you learn how to select packaged foods wisely, you can have your chips and crackers and eat them, too. The key is to trade up in quality by learning to compare the nutritional value of similar packaged foods. In other words, if you feel like eating chips, fine. Eat chips, but choose more nutritious chips.

The Skill: Learning How to Decipher Food Labels Effectively

Choosing healthier foods and getting in the habit of reading nutrition labels can improve your health and help you lose excess pounds. In fact, according to a 2012 study published in *Agricultural Economics*, women who routinely read nutritional labels have a body mass index (BMI) that's on average 1.5 points lower than women who don't read labels.

Making a habit of reading nutrition labels can also naturally improve the quality of your diet. In a study of 1,200 young adults, researchers from the University of Minnesota found that those who reported reading nutrition labels frequently were more likely to have healthier eating habits (in particular, they ate less fast food and added sugar and consumed more fiber, fruits, and vegetables), compared with less-frequent label readers. The surprising part: Those who read nutrition labels frequently tended to have healthier eating habits, even if they didn't believe it's important to prepare healthy meals.

Rule number one: Ignore the claims on the front of a food package. That real estate is owned by the manufacturer, and the wording is designed to make foods sound appealing or healthful, whether or not they actually are, in order to get you to buy them. Instead, turn the package over and look for the Nutrition Facts panel, which is regulated by the Food and Drug Administration (FDA). Start with the serving size and the number of servings in the package, then look at the calories per serving. Use your judgment to determine whether a single serving is realistic for you and whether it's a reasonable calorie bargain, considering the serving size. Next, check the fat information, including the amount of total fat, saturated fat, polyunsaturated fat, monounsaturated fat, and cholesterol, as well as the percentage daily value for each. Your best bet is to choose items that derive no more than 30 percent of their calories from fat, with a maximum of 10 percent from saturated fat. When it comes to sodium, it's generally wise to avoid foods that provide more than 100 milligrams of sodium per 100-calorie serving; this will help you keep your sodium intake within the recommended limit per day. The listings for total carbohydrate and protein are pretty straightforward, but the sugar content is a trickier matter, because it includes both naturally occurring sugar and added sugar. Look at the ingredients list to see if sugar has been added from a source other than the food itself (say, oranges in orange juice). Also, keep in mind: While not more than 10 percent of your daily calories should come from added sugar, no more than 25 percent of your total calories should come from *any* sugar. As far as fiber goes, a food should have at least 2 and preferably 3 grams of fiber per 100-calorie serving.

Next, read the ingredients list. If you can't place the contents of the product in any part of the universe you're familiar with—if it doesn't come from a plant, a mineral, or an animal, for example—you may want to think twice about putting the food in your body. Remember: Ingredients are listed in the order of their quantity within the food, so the higher an ingredient falls on the list, the more of it there is in the product. That's why it's smart to steer clear of foods that have sugar (or honey, cane juice, fruit juice concentrate, syrup of any kind, or anything ending in -*ose*) listed among the first three ingredients. Some pasta sauces have more sugar than chocolate sauce, and some cereals have more salt than potato chips—but there's no good reason for all that sugar or salt to be there. And, as we saw in chapter 6, when there are competing flavors such as sweet and salty in one food item, the combo makes you want to eat more.

Similarly, avoid foods with trans fats or partially hydrogenated oils. I also suggest avoiding artificial ingredients of any kind, sugar substitutes such as aspartame, and monosodium glutamate. In general, if you stick with foods that have ingredients you can recognize and pronounce, and foods that were foods when your grandparents were kids, you can't go too far wrong! Something else to keep in mind: Products that contain multiple grains or that are fortified with vitamins are likely to have longer ingredients lists. In that case, look for the word *artificial* on the list; if it's there, put the item back on the shelf.

Manufacturers often use regulatory loopholes to make you think you're getting something you're not. To become a better-informed shopper, wise up to the real meaning behind these common claims on food labels:

The Claim: Zero Trans Fats

What it really means: To make this claim, a product must contain less than 0.5 grams of trans fats per serving, per FDA guidelines. What manufacturers sometimes do is give the nutritional information for a tiny serving size; that way, there may be less than 0.5 grams of trans fats in the serving specified, but if you end up eating four times that amount—which actually may be a reasonable portion—you'd consume nearly 2 grams of artery-clogging trans fats. If you see "hydrogenated oil," "partially hydrogenated oil," or "shortening" listed in the ingredients, the product contains trans fat, and you'll want to avoid it.

The Claim: Made with Real Fruit

What it really means: There's no official requirement for this phrase. So the entire box of toaster pastries, cereal bars, cookies, fruit leather, or other product could contain mere smidgens of real fruit or drops of fruit juice or fruit extract—and it would be legit for the package to carry this claim. In other words, there's no way to know how much "real fruit" is in it. If fruit is listed among the first three ingredients, that's a good sign, but remember to pay attention to the rest of the nutritional profile.

The Claim: All Natural

What it really means: There are no official guidelines for using this claim on packaged foods—the product could still have added chemicals, including preservatives. So "all natural" is just marketing-speak designed to give the pudding, cereal, ice cream, or other processed food a wholesome image. Plus, it's worth keeping in mind that sugar and butter are natural, so a product that's labeled "all natural" could have heaps of sugar or butter in it, rendering it less than healthy. (When it comes to meat and poultry, the USDA requires that products labeled as "natural" contain no artificial ingredients or added color and be only minimally processed, but they still may contain additives such as broth or other flavor enhancers.) Your best bet is to focus on the food's nutritional value rather than getting hung up on whether it's natural by reading the Nutrition Facts panel and the ingredients list to see if the items you expect to be in the product are among the first listed.

The Claim: Good Source of Fiber

What it really means: To carry this claim, one serving must provide 10 to 19 percent of the recommended daily intake for fiber (2.5 to 4.75 grams per serving), based on a daily meal plan of 2,000 calories. This isn't great, but it's not paltry, either. By contrast, a product can be labeled as "an excellent source of fiber" if it contains 20 percent or more of the recommended daily value. Check the Nutrition Facts panel for the actual amount of fiber in a serving.

The Claim: No Sugar Added

What it really means: No sugar was added during the preparation, cooking, or baking process—but that doesn't mean the food product is low in sugar. After all, fruit juice may have no added sugar but it contains fructose naturally. Keep in mind: 4 grams of sugar equals approximately 1 teaspoon of sugar, so if you choose a cereal that has 16 grams of sugar in a serving, that's like dropping 4 teaspoons of sugar into your bowl. Also, look at the ingredients list to see if a sweetener other than sugar (perhaps honey, cane juice, or corn syrup) was added. Remember: Sugar goes by many other names, and the higher up the sweet stuff appears on the ingredients list, the more sugar the item contains.

The Claim: A Multigrain Product

What it really means: The product contains two or more different grains, such as rice, oats, corn, or wheat. But it doesn't mean they're "whole" grains; they could be refined. Nor will you typically know how much of those grains are in the food. It also doesn't necessarily mean the food is high in fiber. Search for the word *whole*—as in whole wheat, whole oats, and the like—among the first few ingredients on the ingredients list. Also, look for the Whole Grain Stamp of approval (from the Whole Grains Council), which means the product contains at least 8 grams of whole grain in a serving.

The Claim: Low Calorie/Light/Reduced Fat

What it really means: "Low calorie" means the item contains 40 calories or fewer per serving, but the serving size designated by the manufacturer could be the size of a bottle cap, *and* the product could still be high in fat. In real life, you might naturally eat four times that amount. The "light" label, by contrast, could simply mean lighter flavor or color (in the case of olive oil or corn syrup) but the same number of calories as the original—or it could mean "low calorie" or "low fat" (defined as less than 3 grams per serving). If the label says, "reduced fat," that means the peanut butter, soup, or other food contains 25 percent less fat than the original form. For low-calorie claims, figure out whether the serving size is realistic. If it isn't, think about how many calories you'd likely consume from a satisfying portion. With "light" or "reduced-fat" products, make sure you know the trade-offs: Reduced-fat cookies, reduced-fat peanut butter, and reduced-fat salad dressings, for example, often make up for the loss of flavor with added sodium and sugar.

Generally, foods that have relatively short ingredients lists will be more wholesome and have fewer additives such as flavor enhancers, preservatives, dyes, and the like. An exception: Products that contain multiple grains or that are fortified with vitamins are likely to have longer ingredients lists. In that case, look for the word *artificial* on the list; if it's there, put the item back on the shelf. After reviewing the label, jettison products that, given what they are, seem to have excessive amounts of sugar or salt.

The Skill: Finding Ways to Afford Good Nutrition

There's a widespread perception that more nutritious foods cost more, but that isn't necessarily true. In 2011 my research team from the Yale-Griffin Prevention Research Center compared the prices of more and less nutritious foods within given categories in six supermarkets in Jackson County, Missouri. In some categories, such as spreads (e.g., nut butters), the more nutritious, less highly processed items were more expensive. And while more nutritious breads did tend to cost $0.80 more than less nutritious breads, more nutritious cereals typically cost $1.00 less, and more wholesome cookies cost less, too (an average of $0.64 less per package). When we added it all up, it was a wash—choosing more nutritious foods across various categories was likely to have a negligible effect on the total grocery bill.

Second, some of the so-called "expensive" foods (such as fresh produce) are actually a bargain, if you think about what you're getting for your money. They pack a lot more nutrients and healthfulness into every mouthful and dollar spent than anything else in the food supply. In fact, the USDA recently published a study showing exactly this: When food value is measured reasonably, produce is not nearly as expensive as it seems. But these arguments are philosophical in nature; they have to do with how we perceive and measure the value of food.

Remember, too: some of the most nutritious foods on the planet (including many varieties of beans, lentils, and whole grains) are stunningly *inexpensive*. If you learn even a few vegetarian recipes (for soups, stews, salads, or more ambitious ethnic dishes), you can use beans or lentils as an alternative protein source to meat. You will improve the nutritional quality of the meal, and save a lot of money doing it! You can also save money by forgoing soda and sweet drinks, both of which are fairly expensive sources of empty calories, and sticking with plain H_2O instead. If you shop on a budget, as many of us do, compare prices and sizes to find the best values. If you have a recurring ingredient in many of your meals, see if you can find it in the bulk food aisle.

While the most healthful foods are in the produce aisle, produce spoils a lot quicker than processed foods do, and there's a fair amount of variability in taste (whereas you always know exactly what Doritos will taste like). There are delicious peaches and peaches that taste like plastic, and it's very frustrating to spend money on fresh produce only to find out at home that it's tasteless (or worse). There's definitely a learning curve to selecting ripe fruits and vegetables, but once you get the hang of it, you'll be able to consistently bring home tasty, ready-to-eat produce. The key is to buy firm, brightly colored, blemish- and bruise-free vegetables and greens that are crisp and free of brown spots or wilting. With fruits, look for those that are firm, have a good color and smooth skin, and are free of bruises, blemishes and insect holes. If you have any doubts, don't be shy about asking the produce manager for advice about choosing produce that can be hard to judge—especially items such as melons or pineapples.

Your best bet is to buy fruits and vegetables when they're in season, because they tend to cost much less then. (You can also buy berries in the summer and freeze them for later use.) Try to buy from a local farm, vegetable stand, or co-op that ships fresh fruit and vegetables to your home. With these venues, the produce is often of higher quality and fresher because it's local. As with any purchase, it may take you several tries to find the place that provides the best-tasting and highest-quality produce. Remember, too: It's often less expensive to buy frozen fruits and vegetables, and these items are just as nutritious as their fresh counterparts because the items are generally frozen at their peak, just after being picked. Canned fruits and veggies are another affordable option; just be sure to rinse the fruits (since they're often canned in syrup) and the vegetables (which are often immersed in a salty solution) for optimal nutritional value.

The Skill: Raising Nutrition-Savvy Kids

To make healthy eating habits a family affair, it's important to turn kids from part of the problem into part of the solution and get them to work with you instead of against you. And there's something in it for your kids in the short term, not just the long run. When kids consume a healthy breakfast, for example, they score higher on cognitive function tests and report higher energy levels than when they skip breakfast, according to research from Loughborough University in the United Kingdom.

To help them get with the program, take steps to boost your kids' nutritional know-how so they care about nutrition and can help identify better choices. In a world where beloved cartoon characters such as SpongeBob, Scooby Doo, and Alvin and the Chipmunks entice your kids to eat neon-colored snack foods or sugary cereals, it's hard for them to know what's good for them and what's not. They just know what's appealing on a playful or "cool" level. Once you recognize there's a nefarious influence from television and advertising, you'll realize that you probably have to fight against it. Stand firm and draw the line, because children also need healthy foods in their diets, and many of the foods that are marketed to kids are of questionable nutritional value. For example, when researchers from Yale University examined the nutritional quality of 161 cereals that were available in January and February 2006, they found that cereals that were marketed specifically to children were more concentrated sources of calories, sugar, and sodium and contained less fiber and protein than regular cereals. What's more, the majority (66 percent) of the kid-friendly cereals "failed to meet national nutrition standards, particularly with respect to sugar content."

One of my patients, Anna, forty-one, has two kids (ages seven and ten) whom she has struggled to get on board with her attempts to make better food choices for the family. Like most kids, hers are bombarded with commercials for kids' foods on television and online—and naturally they want what they want! Anna initially fought with them over every choice, but frankly, she didn't have the strength for that. So I suggested she try a couple of new tactics.

First, she showed her kids the *Nutrition Detectives* DVD (which I developed), which helped them realize the importance of good foods and took the burden off her to deliver the message. Anna also lives near a supermarket that offers NuVal Scores, so she began taking her kids shopping with her. She'd tell them they could pick out certain crackers, cookies, or cereals, as long as they had a score above a certain number; again, this took the onus off her and put it on the scoring system. The kids simply had to accept the numbers. This two-pronged approach has worked beautifully in enabling Anna to navigate the grocery store with less stress, while upgrading the quality of the entire family's diet. (Those who don't have access to NuVal Scores can use the same principle by designating a certain cutoff for grams of fat or sugar in packaged foods.)

Fortunately, you can make nutritional information tangible and relatable to kids and help them identify healthier choices in surprisingly simple ways. Encourage your children to mute the television when they see commercials, and when they try to get you to buy them unhealthy cereals and snacks in the supermarket, use it as an opportunity to teach them how to be wise shoppers (and make sure no one is hungry when you go shopping). Most kids are naturally curious, and you can capitalize on their inherent curiosity by encouraging them to become supermarket spies, by making a nutrition-detective activity out of reading labels: Encourage kids to investigate whether packaged foods contain the ingredients they should have in them (fruit juice should be made from real fruit, for example, not water and various sweeteners), despite the big, bold claims on the front of the label. Another fun activity is to compare the nutritional benefits of like-minded products (cherries to dried cherries to cherry juice, for example, or grapes to raisins to grape juice). In the produce section, ask them to choose a new fruit or vegetable to try. You can also visit a farmers' market on the weekend to see if you can make some new discoveries together (purple potatoes, anyone?). Then, let them help you prepare a meal with what they chose. This way, they'll have more of an investment in eating healthy foods.

If you have the time and inclination, consider growing some fruits or vegetables in a backyard or community garden. Research from the Mayo Clinic found that when children in fourth through sixth grades participated in garden-based activities twice a week, the vast majority (98 percent!) enjoyed taste-testing fruits and vegetables that were grown, and 91 percent liked learning about the nutritional content of fruits and vegetables. That's a win-win proposition if ever there was one!

You could also set up a contest to motivate everyone in the family to eat more fruits and vegetables. Call it "a rainbow challenge." The goal: to consume as many different colors of fruits and veggies in a day as possible. The prize (besides good health): The winner gets to pick a special weekend activity for the whole family to do together.

The bottom line: If kids want their bodies to perform well and stay healthy, they need to fill them with good-quality fuel in the form of healthy foods in the right amounts. Explain this the right way and kids will get it. After all, they are likely to understand the concept of taking good care of a beloved pet who needs wholesome food to thrive. You might point out that it's the same approach to taking care of their bodies to make sure they continue to run well. It really is that simple.

As a parent of five children, and as an internist who takes care of adults but routinely talks to them about what goes on in their homes, I'm quite familiar with the power the little devils exert on a family's lifestyle habits. When kids just want "the snack with SpongeBob on it," it becomes especially challenging for parents to make their home a safe nutritional environment. On the other hand, when children are motivated to embrace a health-related issue, they can become powerful agents of positive change. Remember: Thanks to public service campaigns aimed at kids and teens, children were the major drivers of increasing seat belt use and fire-safety measures nationwide, and have played a key role in reducing tobacco use among adults. Children can be powerful forces behind positive changes. Sometimes, as parents, we just need to give them a gentle nudge in the right direction. Of course, a robust body of medical literature also tells us what we already know: that moms and dads are important role models for our children. It's no coincidence that children tend to emulate the language we speak, the religion we do or don't practice, and other behaviors. Moreover, the advice to "Do as I say, not as I do" rarely works. If our children respect us, they will do as we do. If they don't respect us—alas, they won't do as we say or as we do. So walk the walk, talk the talk, and eat the right foods.

With teenagers, it's better not to make hard-and-fast rules about food, because that approach tends to backfire. Instead of forbidding fast food or soda, concentrate your efforts on making sure that when they're at home they're eating healthy food; that way, when they go out, they'll have a little leeway and an "unhealthy" meal or snack will not have a major impact. If you control what you can, set a good example, and loosen the reins a bit, you'll build a healthy foundation from which they can launch themselves.

THE DISEASE-PROOF TO-DO LIST:

- Trade up the foods you buy in terms of nutritional value by using the NuVal System or comparing the Nutrition Facts panels and ingredients lists on labels.
- Stock up on healthy staples for your kitchen so you can prepare healthy meals in a flash.
- Develop food label literacy and figure out which packaged foods are worth buying and which aren't.
- Find ways to afford good nutrition by buying produce when it's in season, frozen or canned versions when it's not.
- Make an effort to teach kids about good nutrition by taking them shopping and showing them how to read food labels.

• Eight •

Cooking Healthfully

The Challenge: Relatively few people really know how to cook—or how to cook healthfully—and if they do, they don't always make time for it, given their hectic schedules.

The Right Response: Learn to cook wholesome, nutritious meals by developing the right repertoire, one simple, delicious recipe at a time, and make foods you already like even healthier with some simple adjustments.

The Relevant Skills: Planning your meals ahead of time; putting time on your side when you're super busy; giving recipes a healthier makeover; and steering your family toward healthy eating.

Melanie, a mother of two who runs a non-profit, was in the habit of ordering pizza or takeout meals for her family several nights per week. It was a quick and convenient approach to mealtime, and this way, there were always choices that agreed with everyone. Melanie, fifty-two, is a vegetarian, her eleven-year-old son is a picky eater, and her teenage daughter has a ravenous appetite and wants lots of food to satisfy it. The take-out habit worked for Melanie's work schedule and their busy family life—that is, until Melanie's husband and daughter began complaining about gaining weight and her daughter was found to be gluten-intolerant. Suddenly, Melanie decided she had to find a way to fit healthy dinner preparation into the family's weekday schedule.

She asked friends for recipe recommendations and started with basics—soups, salads, and grains everyone in the family could and would eat. Then she began adding dishes that required minimal assembly—casseroles that included every food group; gluten-free pasta with shrimp, veggies, and tomato sauce; stir-fries made with a variety of vegetables, tofu, and quick-cooking brown rice; and broiled fish with baked potatoes and a leafy green salad. Soon her kids were offering to help, and making weekday dinners became a breeze. Her husband and daughter slimmed down, the family saved money by ordering takeout less frequently, and Melanie felt good knowing they were all eating healthier fare.

The truth is that healthy cooking doesn't have to be a time-consuming, labor-intensive process. In fact, research from UCLA suggests that it takes on average only about ten minutes longer to prepare a wholesome, home-cooked dinner than to serve convenience foods. And if you make enough of the home-cooked stuff so that there are leftovers, you'll be ahead of the game, because you'll actually save time the next day. It costs less than ordering takeout, too! The key is to learn some quick, reliable strategies, so that preparing home-cooked meals will become easier for you. Whether you're new to cooking or you want to upgrade your usual cooking methods to make them healthier, you can learn to prepare tasty, satisfying meals that are good for your health and your waistline—in a matter of minutes.

When it comes right down to it, you can either spend a bit of time now cooking delicious, nutritious meals that you (and your family) can enjoy, or spend days, weeks, or longer on the doctor visits that may become necessary down the road if you develop diabetes, hypertension, heart disease, or other health problems that stem from eating poorly. After all, studies suggest that when people dine out at restaurants, they consume meals with 50 percent more calories, fat, and sodium than when they prepare meals at home. It's also much less expensive to prepare meals at home. While dinner for a family of four at a fast-food chain runs about twenty-eight dollars, preparing a dinner for four of roasted chicken, veggies, salad, and milk costs about half that much. When you look at it from these angles, it's not much of a choice, is it?

Before you can improve your cooking skills, you'll need to ensure you have the right basic equipment on hand to do the job. While there's a seemingly endless supply of kitchen gadgets and gizmos that may seem like a good idea, many aren't necessary. However, there are some essential items you'll need to prepare healthy breakfasts, lunches, and dinners at home. These include sharp knives (at a minimum: a chef's knife, several paring knives, and a serrated bread knife), a vegetable peeler, whisks, cooking brushes, a strainer, measuring spoons, measuring cups, a slotted spoon, wooden spoons, various spatulas, a cheese grater, an instant-read meat thermometer, a steamer, cutting boards, nonstick pans and pots, nonstick baking pans and sheets, roasting pans, a heavy cast-iron grill pan, an electric mixer, a blender, a food processor, and perhaps a crock pot or pressure cooker. This may seem like a hefty list, but you probably have many of these items already.

Once you've stocked up on the basic equipment, it's time to cook! For the sake of your health and waistline, it's far better to bake, sauté, broil, braise, poach, steam, or roast than it is to boil, char, or fry your food. Boiling certain foods (such as vegetables) destroys a higher proportion of nutrients than some of the other techniques. Charring (or blackening) meats, poultry, vegetables, or other foods on a grill can produce carcinogens, so it should be avoided. And frying any food simply adds too much fat. Here's how various healthy cooking methods stack up:

Baking and roasting: Both methods use dry heat in the oven and can be used for cooking fish, poultry, potatoes, casseroles, lasagna, egg dishes, and more. Baking doesn't require adding fat to the food, and with this technique, you avoid charring your food while allowing it to brown on top. With roasting, meat, poultry, or vegetables cook under the oven's dry heat—usually over 400 degrees—so that the outside of the food gets crisp while the inside cooks slowly.

You'll want to use a meat thermometer to make sure meat or poultry is completely cooked through—to an internal temperature of 145 degrees Fahrenheit for steaks and chops, 160 degrees for ground meats, and 165 for poultry.

Braising: A variation on simmering, braising calls for the main ingredient to be browned in butter (which isn't healthy) or olive oil (a healthier choice), then uses liquid—such as water, broth, or wine—to cook the food in an open or covered pan, on the stovetop or in the oven. The cooking liquid keeps everything moist and tender, and the natural juices from the cabbage, pork, chicken, pot roast, or other food adds flavor to the liquid. It's a round robin that leads to a tasty result.

Broiling: With broiling, only a thin layer of air separates the heat source from the steak, chicken, or fish that sits on the broiler pan in your oven. Food cooks quickly on the outside, while allowing the flavor and moistness to be retained inside. Another perk: Broiling allows fat to drip into the pan, rather than be reabsorbed by the food.

Grilling: A relatively quick way to cook meat, poultry, fish, or vegetables, grilling uses direct heat: The food is cooked on a rack above hot coals or a flame, which gives it a smoky flavor and a crisp exterior. As with broiling, fat tends to drip away from the food as it cooks. Just make sure you don't char or blacken the food!

Poaching: With poaching, fish, eggs, or fruit are gently simmered in water, broth, fruit juice, or wine on the stovetop or in the oven until the food becomes tender. Poaching locks in subtle flavors and tenderizes the food as it cooks, without adding fat.

Sautéing and stir-frying: Sautéing involves adding some fat, such as health-promoting olive oil, to a hot pan, then cooking the meat, chicken, or vegetables quickly over direct heat on the stovetop. Using a good-quality nonstick pan will minimize the need for oil.

Stir-frying uses less oil than deep-frying but still allows foods to get browned. Simply heat up a wok or large, deep skillet, drizzle a small amount of olive or sesame oil or spritz some cooking spray into it, turn up the heat on the burner, then add chopped veggies, chunks of chicken or meat, or whatever you want to stir-fry. Keep all the ingredients within reach because the key to stir-frying effectively is to cook the food quickly, continuously moving it around, over high heat.

Steaming: Because it cooks foods over, rather than in, simmering liquid, steaming preserves more of the nutrients and natural texture in foods than boiling does, making it a healthy way to cook fish, poultry, and vegetables fairly quickly. You can use a collapsible steamer insert or a bamboo steamer in an ordinary pot with a top.

From the *Things-You-Never-Knew-You-Never-Knew* Files

Healthy cooking methods have a positive trickle-down effect. Research from the University of Minnesota found that teenagers who engage in food preparation are more likely to enjoy cooking in their mid- to late twenties. Moreover, those who engaged in food preparation between the ages of nineteen and twenty-three typically have healthier diets, including higher intakes of fruits and vegetables and lower intakes of sugar-sweetened beverages and fast food, five years later. So the foundation for lifelong healthy eating for your kids really *can* be set by your habits in the kitchen.

After all, when you cook at home, you're the one who's in control of the ingredients that go into each meal, the cooking methods, and portion sizes. In fact, in a recent study with a group of African American adolescents, researchers from the Johns Hopkins Bloomberg School of Public Health in Baltimore found that having more home-cooked meals didn't necessarily help the teens keep their weight in the normal range.

Only those whose caregivers relied on healthier cooking methods had a reduced risk of being overweight. So the way you cook really *does* matter.

But don't worry: This doesn't mean you have to reinvent the wheel. Breakfast can be easily satisfied with a bowl of whole-grain, high-fiber cold cereal or cooked oatmeal, topped with fresh, dried, or roasted fruits, and skim milk; scrambled eggs (or egg whites), whole-grain toast, and a piece of fruit; or with a cup of nonfat yogurt, whole wheat toast or half a whole-grain bagel topped with all-fruit jam, and a piece of fruit. Add coffee or tea, and you've got a great way to jump-start your day.

Similarly, you can prepare a healthy salad or sandwich to eat at home for lunch—or to take with you to work in an insulated bag with a freezer pack. Still, eating salads can be healthy—or not. Mayonnaise-based salads (such as pasta or potato salad) or salads loaded with cheeses, croutons, bacon bits, and full-fat dressing are not in the healthful zone. Follow this step-by-step system for creating a healthful salad:

Step one: Create a base of greens. Cover your plate or bowl with a variety of lettuces and leafy greens such as arugula, radicchio, mesclun, mizuna, mâche, romaine, watercress, and baby spinach.

Step two: Add chopped fresh veggies (such as cucumbers, red peppers, radishes, carrots, tomatoes, broccoli florets, and the like) to give your salad crunch and volume.

Step three: Choose a source of protein. Add a few tablespoons of chopped hardboiled egg, garbanzo or black beans, cottage cheese, tofu, or up to ½ cup diced cooked chicken, turkey, or shrimp.

Step four: Select a light dressing. Whether you opt for a reduced-fat dressing or oil and vinegar is up to you. Just remember to tread lightly—two tablespoons should be plenty to give you flavor with every forkful.

Use the following guidelines to build a better sandwich—making your favorite lunchtime (or dinnertime) fare healthier, more nutritious, and more satisfying than ever. Pick one item from each category, except the veggies—no limit there!—then assemble your creation.

Bread: Whole-grain bagel, whole-grain roll, whole-grain pita bread, whole-grain bread (2 slices), or a whole wheat tortilla

Spread: Ditch the mayo or butter and choose mustard, hummus, olive or eggplant tapenade, pesto, roasted pepper and white bean puree, mashed avocado, salsa, marinated tofu, or plain nonfat Greek yogurt with herbs and/or shredded cucumber.

Veggies: Lettuce and/or spinach leaves, onions (caramelized or raw), mushrooms, grilled or roasted peppers, grilled eggplant or zucchini, artichoke hearts, tomato or cucumber slices

Protein: Salmon, mahimahi, or veggie burger, marinated tofu, canned salmon or tuna, or a few slices of turkey or chicken (about 2 ounces), egg slices, or low-fat cheese

Come dinnertime, you have two choices. You can think in terms of basic food groups and use the formula outlined in chapter 4: Fill half your plate with vegetables (leafy greens, carrots, zucchini, broccoli, cauliflower, and the like); a quarter with whole grains (such as brown rice, quinoa, or whole-grain pasta) or starchy vegetables (such as corn, peas, potatoes, or root vegetables); and a quarter with lean protein (such as fish, seafood, poultry, pork, tofu, lentils, black beans, or lean beef). Or you can think in terms of preparing multitasking meals that will work for you over the course of several days. Whatever your approach, serve fresh berries or another fruit-based dish for dessert, and voilà!—you've got a full, healthy meal.

The Skill: Planning Your Meals Ahead of Time

Before you head out to do the weekly shopping, spend ten to fifteen minutes planning meals for the week ahead. Think about what you'd like to make for lunches and dinners throughout the week, then create a shopping list with all the ingredients you'll need. Having healthy ingredients readily available makes it that much easier to assemble nutritious dishes at home that will satisfy your hunger. (See chapter 7 for more on this.)

You might prepare some meals ahead of time, helping to streamline your planning and preparation processes for home-cooked meals during a hectic week. And if you make big batches of nutritious staples ahead of time, you can either use them in different ways or divvy them up and freeze them (in dated plastic freezer bags) for later use. A hidden perk: You'll save time cleaning up throughout the week, too. Plus, by having the basis of your meal already prepared, you'll be taking the guesswork out of choosing what to eat and automatically reduce the possibility of choosing something simply because it's quick.

For example, you could prepare a big pot of homemade lentil soup or chili with chicken or vegetable broth, white and black beans, chopped carrots and onions, corn, and stewed tomatoes and divide the portions, freezing some if you'd like. Or, you could use the chili for several meals: Serve it on its own one night—perhaps topped lightly with shredded Monterey Jack cheese or plain nonfat Greek yogurt—over brown rice or whole-grain noodles on another, then drain the liquid and use the chili to make burritos a third night. Similarly, you could roast a large chicken or a turkey: Serve it on its own one night (according to the previously recommended portions), then shred the rest and add it to a homemade soup (with lots of veggies), a stew (with veggies) served over brown rice, or a chili (with kidney beans, corn kernels, and diced tomatoes). The point is to be creative about how to use the base of a meal in numerous ways and let it multitask for you in a healthful, time-saving manner.

You can also use a simple formula for meal planning that works for pasta and casserole-type dishes. Consider what's on the base, what's in the middle layer, and what sauces or other toppings you'll include. First, pick the type of pasta you want to use (whole wheat pasta, whole-grain pasta, or spelt, buckwheat, or kamut pasta); next, choose a few toppings you want to include (perhaps artichoke hearts, roasted bell peppers, roasted eggplant, fresh tomatoes, leeks, sautéed mushrooms, olives and capers, spinach, sun-dried tomatoes, sautéed or roasted zucchini, cannellini beans, seafood, chicken, lean ground beef or turkey); and finally, select your sauce (whether it's marinara sauce, olive oil and garlic, or basil pesto). When you put the pieces together, you've got a healthy meal!

The Skill: Putting Time on Your Side When You're Super Busy

You can take several shortcuts to healthy eating. With a precooked rotisserie chicken (skin removed), shredded low-fat cheese, whole-grain tortillas, precut frozen veggies, and canned beans—you'll have everything you need to "assemble" fajitas at home. Or you could toss that cut-up chicken onto a salad (see salad-building tips just given) and call it a meal. Throw together a quick stir-fry with (defrosted) frozen shrimp, edamame, other veggies, and precooked brown rice. Or you could make a one-dish meal—such as an omelet of eggs, skim milk, spinach, (defrosted) frozen peppers and onions, and low-fat cheese.

For something completely different, you can also combine cooking with socializing by taking turns having healthy potluck meals with your friends and family. The idea: Each of you brings a healthy dish to share, and leftovers are divided among the guests. Along with good food, you can enjoy one another's company, swap recipes, and encourage one another to keep on eating the healthy way. It's positive reinforcement, healthy nutrition, and a good time all rolled into one experience.

The Skill: Giving Recipes a Healthy Makeover

Whenever possible, opt for ingredients that are close to nature (such as fruits, vegetables, and whole grains) instead of using more processed items. Anything packaged should be low in saturated fat, salt, and added sugars. Including fruits, vegetables, and whole grains will also help you pump up the volume of your food, helping you feel fuller and more satisfied from a smaller amount. You can also upgrade the nutritional value of meals you prepare by using skim milk instead of whole milk in your cooking and replacing some (or all) of the all-purpose flour with whole wheat flour, oatmeal, or wheat germ when making breads, muffins, or other baked goods.

Making healthy ingredient substitutions allows you to maintain the familiar taste and appearance of your favorite dishes while boosting their nutritional value and health benefits. Opting for the more nutritious choice can have a variety of trickle-down benefits for your health and waistline. For example, a study from Navarra, Spain, found that when people were assigned to follow a Mediterranean diet that was rich in virgin olive oil for three years, they achieved significantly higher levels of antioxidants in their blood, which was associated with reductions in body weight during that time. In a previous study, this same group of researchers found that sticking with a diet rich in virgin olive oil for three years could reverse the effects of the -174G/C polymorphism of the IL6 gene, which influences levels of systemic inflammation and insulin resistance; both are risk factors for diabetes and heart disease. (Remember: We each have different versions of the same genes; these are referred to as polymorphisms.) The findings in this particular study are yet another example of how we can alter the behavior of our genes at the molecular level by what we do with our forks.

Meanwhile, culinary herbs and spices can give our health a boost as well as infusing our meals with extra flavor. For example, cinnamon may lower blood sugar as well as artery-clogging LDL cholesterol and total cholesterol. Rosemary has strong antioxidant properties and anti-inflammatory effects, both of which can help protect against heart disease and cancer. (Ground cloves, oregano, ginger, allspice, and cinnamon also have been found to have high levels of antioxidant activity.) Thyme, rosemary, and sage can inhibit the growth of human colon cancer cells, according to laboratory research from the University of Georgia. And turmeric (used in Indian curries and stews) has been found to have strong anti-inflammatory properties and appears to inhibit the growth of cancer cells. Moreover, in a recent study from China, curcumin (the major component of turmeric) was found to increase the level of apoptosis (cellular suicide or self-destruction) in triple-negative breast cancer cells in a laboratory setting, thereby inhibiting the cancer cells' growth. (It has been found to have similar effects on lung cancer, prostate cancer, colorectal cancer, and oral cancer cells.)

Here are some smart ingredient swaps worth making:

- Instead of adding butter to a pan before cooking, a light spray of heart-healthy olive oil or canola oil will usually do the trick and prevent food from sticking to the pan. You can also sauté vegetables, poultry, and meat in fat-free broth or wine instead of using butter.

- When recipes call for butter, you can often substitute healthy oils such as olive or canola oil (for main dishes); or you can swap applesauce, pureed prunes, or yogurt for up to half the butter or shortening in many baked goods recipes. This way, your baked goods will stay moist but you can skim off some of the fat. Use nonfat plain Greek yogurt in place of sour cream in recipes, and skim buttermilk or a roux (made up of an olive oil/flour paste whisked with hot milk or broth) instead of cream. In place of cream cheese in baked goods, you can often use a combination of part-skim ricotta cheese and reduced-fat cream cheese.

- Instead of marinating meat, poultry, or fish in an oil-based mixture, use a citrus marinade or low-fat, low-sodium chicken, beef, or vegetable broth with fresh or dried herbs. Marinating tenderizes the meat, reducing the need to add fat during the cooking process.

- Expand your spice and herb repertoire to enhance the flavor of main dishes without using salt. Try sage, thyme, tarragon, basil, chives, oregano, rosemary, minced onion or garlic, and cilantro; ginger, turmeric, cumin, paprika, cinnamon, and cloves; and vinegars, low-sodium soy sauce, citrus juices or grated zest, horseradish, mustards, salsas, or wine, individually or in combinations.

From the *Things-You-Never-Knew-You-Never-Knew* Files

Cooking at home could enhance your lifespan. After following a group of 1,888 men and women over age sixty-five, researchers found that people who cook up to five times a week were 47 percent more likely to still be alive after ten years, according to a 2012 study in *Public Health Nutrition*.

The Skill: Steering Your Family Toward Healthy Eating

Conflicting food preferences within your family can make improving your dietary pattern considerably more challenging, especially if you're sharing meals with family members every day. If you don't engage your family in a healthful way of eating, you may eventually feel as if you're left with only two choices: to abandon your efforts or to eat differently from the rest of your family, neither of which is a viable option for the long haul.

A patient of mine named Carla, thirty-eight, found this to be true. After having three children, she was carrying an extra 30 pounds and she wanted to slim down. For a while, she did quite well on Weight Watchers, which I consider a very good, responsible weight-loss program, but there was a problem: She was on the Weight Watchers program alone. Her husband wasn't on it. Her kids weren't on it. So she still came home to a vast array of nutritionally questionable foods, from cheese puffs to chips to gummy bears. In Carla's case, the temptations of readily accessible, tasty junk foods won out over her own diet plan, and she found herself going off the reservation and gaining, not losing, weight.

To me, the solution was obvious: Ditch the junk. But while that's a simple concept, the execution can be hard, because it often means getting the whole family on board. Carla and I worked on tackling this together. She talked to her kids (ages six, eight, and ten) about why eating healthier foods was important for them all, and talked to her husband about not only taking better care of himself but also helping Carla reclaim the health and appearance she wanted. Carla helped her family realize that helping one another be healthy was a good way of demonstrating love. And with their help, she found the strength to reach her weight goals—and the goal of treating her family to a healthier diet.

Rather than catering to the lowest common denominator (otherwise known as the picky eater in the family), enlist the support and participation of your family in improving eating habits for the entire family. Family is (or should be) about shared love and shared responsibility, and for both reasons, family members should be engaged in any effort toward a challenging change, whether it's to lose weight or find better health through good nutrition. Enlisting the support of your family will make you stronger and far more able to achieve lasting success in either respect. Plus, you love them and want to share with them the benefits of the healthy changes you're making.

So tell family members plainly, "I love you, and I need you. I want to be healthy, and I'm doing something about it. So please help me make the transition to better eating habits and to fitting physical activity into each day. And since I love you and want you to be healthy, let me help you do the same. Let's do this together." This conversation can be spouse to spouse, or parent to child, or in the setting of a family meeting. You can choose the words and the timing that best suit the relationship(s).

After this initial conversation, it's best to back off a bit. Let your family know that this won't involve a sudden, radical overhaul of the family diet and that you don't plan to become the nutrition police. Make a commitment to plan a healthful diet together and identify dietary changes that the family is most willing to make, and adopt those first. Let everyone know that adjusting to new, more healthful foods will require a transition period of one to two weeks. Then take the wheel and drive the bus in a healthier direction. Use the skills you've learned so far to make more healthful versions of your family's favorite dishes, snacks, or desserts, and compromise on must-have foods. When you handle it this way, you may find that your request for their encouragement and participation probably won't invite much opposition.

If your children balk at new recipes, rest assured: They won't let themselves starve. Their taste buds will grow accustomed to the newer fare. In the meantime, it's up to you to serve the healthy meals you want your family to enjoy, and it's up to each family member to decide how much to eat. Cajoling, bribing, or bargaining with children to "have just two more bites" or to "clean your plate" are common practices among parents, but these can backfire, causing your children to lose touch with their bodies' natural signals of hunger and fullness. When researchers at the University of California, San Francisco, observed dinnertime dynamics among 142 families of kindergartners, they found that 85 percent of parents encouraged children to eat more and 83 percent of the kids did consume more than they would have naturally; 38 percent ate quite a bit more than they might have otherwise. The problem is that this sort of pressure disrupts the natural satiety signals in the children's bodies and inadvertently promotes overeating.

It's also best to use nonfood rewards with children so they don't develop a habit of eating for emotional reasons. Instead of using food to show love or lavish praise on your children, give them extra one-on-one time with you—by taking them on a special bike ride, an outing to the zoo, or another treat that involves time well spent.

Eating a wholesome diet is a behavior like any other: It must be taught and practiced, again and again, by everyone. When researchers from the University of Newcastle in Australia surveyed nearly four hundred parents of preschoolers about the home food environment and their children's fruit and vegetable intake, they found a strong association between kids' fruit and vegetable consumption and their parents' intake; moreover, the more often parents provided their child with fruit and vegetables each day, the more produce the young kids ate on a daily basis. So don't underestimate the power of parental modeling or repeated exposure to healthy foods!

Once these wholesome eating habits take root, they have a better chance of thriving and becoming sustainable for the whole family. The best way to get there is together. When researchers from the University of Minnesota tracked the eating habits of 677 adolescents from middle school through high school, they found that the teens who had regular family meals over the five-year period had higher daily intakes of vegetables, fiber, vitamins (such as A, B_6, and folate), and minerals (including calcium, magnesium, potassium, iron, and zinc) than their peers who had less frequent family meals. In other words, sharing regular family meals when your kids are in early adolescence can help them maintain healthier eating habits when they reach their late teens.

Food for Thought, Thoughts for Food

Whether you want to learn how to cook healthfully or you simply want to broaden your repertoire, it pays to invest in some good cookbooks. Weekends are a great time to peruse recipes and perhaps cook one or two meals ahead of time to make the coming week easier. Here are several cookbooks worth checking out:

Cooking Light: The Essential Dinner Tonight Cookbook, by the editors of Cooking Light magazine

How to Cook Everything: Simple Recipes for Great Food, by Mark Bittman

Moosewood Restaurant Cooks at Home: Fast and Easy Recipes for Any Day, by The Moosewood Collective

Moosewood Restaurant Low-Fat Favorites: Flavorful Recipes for Healthful Meals, by The Moosewood Collective

Quick & Healthy Recipes and Ideas: For People Who Say They Don't Have Time to Cook Healthy Meals, by Brenda Ponichtera

(continued)

The Supermarket Diet Cookbook, by Janis Jibrin and Susan West-moreland

The Volumetrics Eating Plan: Techniques and Recipes for Feeling Full on Fewer Calories, by Barbara Rolls

Weight Watchers New Complete Cookbook

Cooking well doesn't have to be an elaborate affair. You can keep it simple and healthy and still create delicious meals and a pleasant dining experience. With regular practice, planning and cooking nutritious meals will become second nature to you. You'll become more efficient in the kitchen, and your taste buds will likely develop a preference for your own healthful fare. Cooking healthfully will become the new normal for you, which is just as it should be.

Now that you've learned how to reshape your plate, choose healthy ingredients, and conceptualize health-promoting meals, here are some of our favorite nutritious, delicious recipes to help you get started experimenting in the kitchen. Think of this as a way to kick it off in the right direction, from morning 'til night. You've already learned how to build a better salad and sandwich—both are great options for packed lunches for yourself or your kids. Here are a few breakfast suggestions, ten main meals (many of which reflect the Mediterranean style of eating) for dinner or lunch, and a few desserts.

Almond Banana Smoothie

Serves 1

⅓ ripe banana
1 teaspoon natural almond butter or unsalted peanut butter
2 tablespoons fat-free vanilla yogurt
2 tablespoons fat-free powdered milk
⅓ cup skim milk
½ cup ice

Place all ingredients in a blender and process until smooth. (Note: Recipe can be doubled, tripled, or quadrupled to serve more people.)

Cinnamon French Toast with Sliced Strawberries

Serves 1

 1 egg
 ½ cup skim milk
 ½ teaspoon ground cinnamon
 2 slices whole-grain bread
 Canola oil cooking spray
 ½ cup strawberries, washed and sliced

Heat a nonstick skillet large enough to hold both pieces of bread over medium heat. Whisk the egg, milk, and cinnamon in a shallow bowl. Dip the bread in the egg mixture, coating both sides lightly. Lightly coat the hot pan with the cooking spray, then add the bread, cooking for 1–2 minutes, before flipping bread over and cooking for another minute. Top with sliced strawberries and serve. (Note: Recipe can be doubled, tripled, or quadrupled to serve more people.)

Red Pepper and Cheese Omelet

Serves 1

 Olive oil cooking spray
 2 large eggs
 2 tablespoons skim milk
 Pinch of herbs (such as thyme, basil, or parsley)
 2 ounces diced roasted red peppers
 1 tablespoon shredded part-skim mozzarella cheese

Lightly coat a nonstick skillet with olive oil spray and place over medium heat. In a small bowl, whisk the eggs, milk, and herbs. Pour the egg mixture into the hot skillet. As it begins to set, gently lift the edges with a spatula and tilt the pan so the uncooked mixture flows around the cooked. Continue until the mixture no longer runs freely in the pan. Spoon the peppers and cheese onto one half of the omelet, then fold it over and cook on both sides until golden. Serve with whole-grain toast.

Baked Fish with Tomatoes, Olives, and Capers

Serves 4

> 1½ pounds tilapia fillets or tuna steaks
> ¼ teaspoon salt
> 1 can (15 ounces) diced tomatoes with their own juice
> 2 tablespoons tomato paste
> 2 tablespoons water
> ½ cup kalamata olives, chopped
> 2 tablespoons capers
> 2 tablespoons sun-dried tomatoes, drained and julienned
> 1 tablespoon extra-virgin olive oil
> 4 cloves garlic, peeled and thickly sliced
> 6 cornichons (optional)
> Fresh ground pepper to taste

Preheat oven to 375°F. Rinse and pat dry the fish then lightly salt both sides. Place remaining ingredients in a baking pan and stir to blend. Add the fish to the baking pan and spoon some of the sauce on top. Bake for 20–30 minutes (until fish is cooked through), basting with pan juices once or twice during cooking.

Shrimp Stir-Fry with Veggies, Garlic, Ginger, and Peanuts

Serves 4

40 frozen (about 1 pound) medium shrimp (raw), peeled and
   deveined
½ cup roasted unsalted peanuts
1½ tablespoons peanut oil
2 cloves garlic, minced
2 teaspoons minced fresh ginger
½ cup diced yellow onion
½ cup diced red bell pepper
½ cup diced snow peas
½ cup diced mushrooms
4 tablespoons low-sodium soy sauce
2 tablespoons lime juice
12 ounces bean sprouts, rinsed
2 scallions, cut into 1-inch pieces

Quickly defrost the shrimp by rinsing them in cold water. Pat them
dry with paper towel and set them aside. Place peanuts in a mini food
processor and grind them into a coarse meal; set aside. Heat peanut oil
in a wok (or large frying pan) over medium-high heat until it is just
about to smoke, then add the garlic and ginger, stirring for about 30 seconds. Add the shrimp, onion, pepper, peas, and mushrooms and cook
for 3–4 minutes, until the shrimp is cooked through. Add the soy sauce
and lime juice and continue stirring and tossing until all the ingredients
are mixed together. Mix in about ⅔ of the ground peanuts, plus the bean
sprouts and scallion, cook for 2–3 minutes more, and then remove from
heat. Top with the rest of the ground peanuts and serve.

Dijon Chicken Salad

Serves 4

> 4 chicken breast cutlets (3 ounces each), grilled or baked, then diced
> 1 cup diced sweet red bell pepper
> ⅛ cup chopped walnuts
> 2½ tablespoons fat-free plain Greek yogurt
> 4 teaspoons Dijon mustard
> 4 teaspoons olive oil
> 2 teaspoons cider vinegar
> Pinch of garlic powder
> Pinch of salt
> Freshly ground pepper to taste

Combine all ingredients in a small bowl. Chill until you're ready to serve.

Pasta e Fagioli with Spinach Marinara Sauce

Serves 4

> 1 tablespoon extra-virgin olive oil
> 4 garlic cloves, minced
> 12 ounces raw baby spinach, rinsed
> 1 (28-ounce) can crushed tomatoes (no added oil or sugar)
> 1 (15-ounce) can cannellini beans, well rinsed and drained
> ½ cup kalamata olives
> 1 bay leaf
> 1 teaspoon dried thyme leaves
> ¼ teaspoon salt
> Fresh ground pepper to taste
> 12 ounces whole wheat organic penne with milled flaxseed

Heat the olive oil over medium heat in a large pan. Add the garlic and sauté for a few seconds. Add the spinach in bunches and cook until it is completely wilted, about 4–5 minutes. Add the remaining ingredients except the pasta and simmer, uncovered, for 8–10 minutes. In the meantime, cook the penne according to the package directions. Drain the pasta well and divide into four servings, topping with the sauce.

Stuffed Mexican Bell Peppers

Serves 4

4 red or yellow bell peppers (pick short, stout ones that will stand upright)
2 teaspoons olive oil
1 clove garlic, minced
½ pound lean ground turkey breast
1 (15-ounce) can fat-free refried beans
1½ cups mild salsa
¾ cup cooked bulgur wheat (cook according to package directions)
¼ cup shredded part-skim mozzarella cheese

Preheat oven to 350°F. Wash and dry the peppers, then slice off the tops, removing core and seeds. Place them in a baking pan, standing up, and set aside. Heat olive oil in a pan over medium heat. Add the garlic and sauté for a few seconds, then add the turkey and brown thoroughly, stirring often, about five to ten minutes. Add the refried beans, salsa, and cooked bulgur wheat, mix, and continue to cook for a few minutes until the mixture gets bubbly. Divide the stuffing among the peppers, topping each with cheese. Bake for 20–25 minutes then place under the broiler just until the cheese is sizzling and golden, about 5 minutes.

Lentil and Kale Soup

Serves 4

>   2 teaspoons olive oil
>   1 large onion, chopped
>   1 garlic clove, minced
>   1 cup chopped carrots
>   1 cup diced sweet red bell pepper
>   2 cups low-sodium chicken or vegetable broth
>   1 cup dried lentils, rinsed
>   2 cups water
>   1 cup shredded kale leaves (tough stems removed), or baby spinach
>   1 (14.5-ounce) can fire-roasted diced tomatoes (no salt added),
>   drained
>   ½ teaspoon ground cumin
>   ¼ teaspoon salt
>   Freshly ground pepper to taste
>   2 teaspoons fresh lemon juice

In a large nonstick pot, heat the olive oil over medium heat. Sauté the onion, garlic, carrots, and red pepper until soft, about 5–7 minutes. Add the broth, lentils, and water and bring to a boil. Reduce heat and let it simmer, covered, until the lentils are tender, about 45 minutes. Add kale, tomatoes, cumin, salt, and pepper, and cook, stirring occasionally, until the kale softens, about 5 minutes. Stir in the lemon juice, adjust seasonings to taste, and serve.

Pesto Shrimp and Pasta Primavera

Serves 4

40 frozen (about 1 pound) medium shrimp, raw
2 tablespoons grated Parmesan or pecorino cheese
2 cups (packed) fresh basil leaves
3 tablespoons pine nuts
2 cloves garlic
¼ teaspoon salt
⅓ cup extra-virgin olive oil, plus 1 tablespoon reserved
10 ounces organic whole wheat rotini pasta with flaxseed
Olive oil spray
1 (16-ounce) bag frozen (or about 2 cups fresh) chopped vegetables
   (broccoli, carrots, peppers, etc.)

Quickly defrost the shrimp in cold water. Peel them and pat dry with paper towel; set aside. Place the cheese, basil, pine nuts, garlic, and salt in a food processor, mixing until everything is blended together. Scrape down the sides of the bowl. Add ⅓ cup olive oil to mixture and pulse until incorporated. Cover and refrigerate. Cook the pasta according to the package directions, then drain and rinse in cold water. While the pasta is cooking, lightly spray a cast-iron grill pan with the olive oil spray and place over high heat. When the pan is very hot, add the shrimp and grill for 2–3 minutes on each side. Do not overcook. Set the shrimp aside in a large serving bowl. Add remaining 1 tablespoon olive oil to the same pan and sauté the veggies for a few minutes until they're heated through. Mix the pasta, veggies, and pesto into the bowl with the shrimp, stirring to blend evenly before serving.

Grilled Chicken with Caramelized Onions and Sun-Dried Tomatoes on Whole Wheat Pita

Serves 4

> 2 tablespoons extra-virgin olive oil
> 1¼ pounds raw boneless, skinless chicken breasts
> ¼ teaspoon salt
> 2 yellow onions, thinly sliced
> ½ cup sun-dried tomatoes
> Olive oil cooking spray
> Freshly ground black pepper
> 4 large whole wheat pitas
> Mixed greens of your choice

Heat the oil in a medium nonstick skillet over medium heat. Rinse the chicken, pat dry and lightly salt; set aside. When the skillet is hot, add the onion and a pinch of salt, then cook for 10 minutes, covered, stirring occasionally. Add the sun-dried tomatoes to the onion and cook for an additional 10 minutes, until the onions are soft and have turned golden brown. While the onions are cooking, heat a large cast-iron grill pan over medium-high heat. Lightly coat the pan with the cooking spray and then grill the chicken breasts for 6–8 minutes on each side, adding the ground pepper to taste. Remove the cooked chicken to a cutting board and slice into strips. To serve, place a whole pita on each plate, and top with equal portions of the mixed greens, chicken, and onion-tomato mixture.

Spinach Salad with Lentils, Feta, and Walnuts

Serves 4

4 teaspoons Dijon mustard

8 teaspoons vinegar

8 teaspoons olive oil

4 tablespoons water

Salt and freshly ground pepper to taste

8 cups fresh baby spinach leaves, rinsed

1⅓ cup cooked lentils (cook according to package directions)

4 tablespoons chopped walnuts

2½ tablespoons crumbled feta cheese

Place the mustard, vinegar, oil, water, salt, and pepper in a small bowl and whisk to blend. In a large bowl, toss the spinach leaves with the lentils. Pour the dressing over the spinach and lentils and toss well. Sprinkle with the walnuts and feta.

Orange Sesame Tuna

Serves 4

4 tuna steaks (4 ounces each)

⅓ cup sesame seeds

2 tablespoons organic whole wheat pastry flour (or oat bran flour)

¼ teaspoon garlic powder

Pinch of salt and of freshly ground pepper

2 tablespoons sesame oil

¾ cup orange juice

1 tablespoon orange juice concentrate (Note: You can use the leftover concentrate to make orange juice)

1 tablespoon low-sodium soy sauce

1 tablespoon honey

1 teaspoon minced fresh ginger

Preheat the oven to 400ºF. Rinse the tuna steaks and pat them dry. Combine the sesame seeds with the flour, garlic powder, salt, and pepper. Dredge one side of each tuna steak in the sesame seed–flour mixture. Heat the oil over high heat in an ovenproof nonstick pan. When the pan is hot, place the tuna steaks sesame-side down and sear for 2–3 minutes. Turn the steaks over and transfer the pan into the preheated oven for 6–8 minutes, until the steaks look cooked on the outside. While the tuna continues to cook in the oven, mix the orange juice, juice concentrate, soy sauce, honey, and ginger in a small saucepan and bring the mixture to a boil. Reduce the heat and simmer the sauce for 3–4 minutes until it thickens. Spoon sauce over the tuna and serve.

Peach Almond Cobbler

Serves 4

> 1 teaspoon regular Smart Balance spread

FILLING:

> 6 cups sliced fresh ripe peaches (about 9 medium unpeeled peaches)
> 2 tablespoons brown sugar
> ½ teaspoon cinnamon
> ⅛ teaspoon almond extract
> 1 tablespoon whole wheat pastry flour

TOPPING:

> ½ cup almond meal*
> ½ cup whole wheat pastry flour
> ½ cup rolled oats
> 3 tablespoons brown sugar
> 2 tablespoons regular Smart Balance spread
> 1 tablespoon fat-free buttermilk

Preheat oven to 400°F. Spread 1 teaspoon Smart Balance spread onto the bottom of a 9-inch pie dish. Mix filling ingredients together in a bowl then pour mixture into pie dish. Set aside. Combine topping ingredients in a bowl, working the mixture with your fingers until it is crumbly. Sprinkle it evenly over the filling. Bake for 15–20 minutes, until the top is golden and the juices are sizzling.

*To make almond meal, pulse unsalted almonds in a food processor, but be careful not to overdo it or you will end up with almond butter.

Zucchini Bread

Serves 8 to 10, depending on thickness of the slices

   3 cups whole wheat pastry flour
   2 teaspoons baking powder
   3 teaspoons ground cinnamon
   3 large eggs
   1 cup canola oil
   1½ cups white sugar
   2 teaspoons vanilla extract
   3 cups grated zucchini (about 3 medium zucchini, unpeeled)
   1 cup chopped walnuts (optional)

Grease and flour two 8-by-4-inch loaf pans. Preheat oven to 325°F. Sift flour, baking powder, and cinnamon together in a bowl. In another large bowl, beat eggs, oil, sugar, and vanilla. Add dry ingredients to the wet mixture and beat well. Stir in the grated zucchini and the walnuts, if using, until well combined. Pour batter into prepared pans. Bake for 45–50 minutes, or until a toothpick inserted in the center comes out clean. Cool in pan for 20 minutes, then remove loaves to a rack and cool completely before serving.

Mexican Chocolate Cake

   2¼ cups whole wheat pastry flour

   ¾ cup unsweetened Dutch process cocoa powder

   2 teaspoons baking powder

   1 teaspoon ground cinnamon

   3 large eggs

   1 cup canola oil

   1¾ cups white sugar

   2 teaspoons vanilla extract

   3 cups grated zucchini (about 3 medium zucchini)

Preheat oven to 325°F. Grease and flour a Bundt pan and set aside. Sift together flour, cocoa powder, baking powder, and cinnamon in a bowl and set aside. Beat eggs, oil, sugar, and vanilla together in a large bowl with an electric mixer. Add dry ingredients to the wet mixture and beat well. Stir in zucchini and any zucchini juice with a silicone spatula until well combined. Pour batter into the prepared pan. Bake for about 45–50 minutes, or until a toothpick inserted in the center comes out clean. Cool in pan for at least 20 minutes before removing and serving.

THE DISEASE-PROOF TO-DO LIST:

- Get in the habit of planning meals ahead of time so you can be sure to have ingredients available when you need them.
- Build healthier, more satisfying salads and sandwiches by taking a layered approach.
- Use meal preparation shortcuts when you're especially busy, such as choosing canned or frozen veggies, marinated tofu, rotisserie chicken, and other precooked ingredients.
- Give recipes a nutritional makeover by using healthy oils instead

of butter, nonfat Greek yogurt instead of sour cream, and broths, herbs, and spices instead of heavy sauces.

- Get family members invested in developing healthier eating habits by finding ways to manage food conflicts or making healthier versions of your family's favorite foods.

• Nine •

Taking Your Eating Habits on the Road

The Challenge: In many cultures around the world today, eating is done primarily at home, so food exists in a controlled environment. We're a society that's on the move, which means many of our meals are prepared by other people.

The Right Response: We don't control the weather, but we can carry an umbrella and wear a raincoat. Plan for your meals the way you would prepare for rain.

The Relevant Skills: Taking control of your eating habits at work; developing a personal food policy for eating out; decoding restaurant menus; questioning your server and making healthy requests; maintaining control of your eating and drinking while socializing; standing up to food pushers; and sidestepping sabotage or turning it into support.

There's a famous restaurant scene in the movie *When Harry Met Sally*. I'm not talking about "I'll have what she's having!" I'm referring to the one early in the movie where Sally (played by Meg Ryan) and Harry (played by Billy Crystal) are having lunch at a diner while driving from the University of Chicago to New York City. Harry orders the "number three," while Sally, a persnickety eater, begins customizing her lunch order, asking for a chef salad with oil and vinegar on the side, followed by apple pie à la mode with the pie heated but with strawberry ice cream instead of vanilla and whipped cream, but only if it's real, and if it's not then she doesn't want any of it. At this, Harry engages in a serious bout of eye rolling, and as viewers, we share his exasperation.

After watching Sally do this routine many times over the next ten years, Harry comments, "*On the side* is a very big thing for you." To which Sally responds, "I just want it the way I want it!" The truth is that we should all have more Sally moments when we're dining out. As long as they're in the spirit of making healthier choices at restaurants, they could help each of us protect our health and our waistlines.

Once upon a time, and not that long ago, eating out was often reserved for special occasions—it was a chance for a treat, a splurge, or simply a culinary adventure of some sort. Sometimes it still is. But these days many people eat out at restaurants, the office, other people's homes, or on the fly several times each week. It's become part of our lifestyle. And here's the reality: If you eat out often, restaurant foods, takeout foods, or cafeteria fare will have a large impact on your dietary intake—both the calories you consume and the nutrients that come with them—for better or for worse.

Unfortunately, the "for worse" effect often predominates, but it doesn't have to be this way. In a study involving nearly twenty-three hundred men and women in their twenties, researchers at the University of Minnesota found that those who went to fast-food restaurants more frequently had a higher risk of being overweight or obese, and they consumed more sugar-sweetened beverages and fat and more calories overall than at full-service restaurants. (By contrast, those who went to full-service restaurants tended to consume more vegetables.) Indeed, numerous studies have suggested that people who eat fast food frequently are at higher risk of obesity. The correlation is hardly surprising, given that fast food tends to be high in calories, relatively nutritionally poor, and high in salt, fat, and sugar, all of which stimulate appetite.

The concern isn't just a matter of weight; it's a matter of health as well. When someone else is preparing your food, and you don't know what's in it, your health is basically at the mercy of the cook's or chef's culinary practices. No wonder research from Australia found that young women who ate carryout food twice a week or more had considerably higher fasting blood sugar and insulin levels—both are risk factors for diabetes and heart disease—than those who got carryout less often.

Preventing such negative effects while eating out requires attention to detail and savvy ordering skills. You can use the same skills you've been learning to apply to your food choices at home to choosing nutritionally balanced meals at restaurants. While the more leisurely pace of restaurant dining means you'll have more time to savor the flavors and to sample different dishes, it also means there will be more time for the restaurant's ambience to influence your eating habits as you sit at the table.

One of my patients, Ben, a forty-five-year-old sales executive, learned this the hard way. About a year ago, he came to see me for a general checkup and some weight-loss advice. Over the previous five years, Ben had gained 25 pounds and he was at a loss as to how it had happened. As we discussed his lifestyle, the explanation became fairly obvious: increases in his demands at work meant less time for basketball or going to the gym, and more time spent traveling for business and eating out with clients. Ben mostly had restaurant food to thank for his weight gain.

Fortunately, this was a fairly easy problem to solve. After that appointment, he made a habit of starting each meal with a mixed green salad (light on the dressing), limiting the amount of bread he ate, asking about how dishes were prepared, and slowing down his alcohol intake. He also began skipping dessert more often. Meanwhile, at home, he and his wife took steps to improve the nutritional quality of their meals, and Ben made exercise a priority again. The last time I saw him, he was down 18 of those 25 pounds and feeling great!

His experience is hardly unusual. According to research at the University of Pittsburgh, cutting back on eating at restaurants was a key factor in helping overweight and obese women lose weight in the first six months of weight loss; however, by forty-eight months, it was no longer as influential. By then, decreasing consumption of desserts, sugar-sweetened beverages, and meats and cheeses, and increasing consumption of fruits and vegetables had become more important influences.

As a starting point, skip restaurants that offer buffets or all-you-can-eat options. Buffets activate our inclination to overindulge, and they play to our vulnerability to sensory-specific satiety. (See chapter 6 for a refresher on this.) If you find yourself unable to avoid the buffet, decide ahead of time what and how much you'll eat and abide by your decision. Start with a salad or grilled or roasted vegetables to help you fill up, and avoid concentrated sources of fat and calories such as cheeses, processed meats, and creamy or buttery dishes.

The Skill: Taking Control of Your Eating Habits at Work

At work, you may feel like a victim of circumstance as far as your eating habits go. As we've seen, research shows that we tend to eat more food if it is readily available, when there's a greater variety to choose from, and when we have easy access to it. So when a tray of cookies is sitting on the conference room table during a meeting, or a bowl of candy is always filled to capacity on a colleague's desk, it can be difficult to resist. (By the way, you might consider whose hands have been in that bowl and where those hands have been. I'm just sayin'.) Think of it this way: you don't let anyone else decide what you'll wear on a given day or whether to take an umbrella if it looks like rain, so why would you let someone else decide what you should eat?

The ideal solution would be to involve your entire office in the quest to replace unhealthy snack options with healthier ones, such as a bowl of fresh fruit or fruit salad or a platter of raw vegetables and hummus, salsa, or guacamole. Try to work within your organization's management structure—many employers will welcome the chance to improve the health of their employees, since healthy employees will cost them less in health care costs and absenteeism in the long term.

If you can't succeed on that front, keep a stash of healthy snacks in your own desk—packaged instant (plain) oatmeal and small bags of dried cranberries or raisins and chopped walnuts; homemade energy mix with dried cherries, apricots, nuts, and a whole-grain cereal; or portable fruits such as apples, bananas, or clementines. (See the box "Snacking Tips" for more great snacking ideas.) This way, you can take a preemptive strike against hunger before meetings or bring your own healthy snack to the table; you'll also be less likely to dip into the communal candy dish. These healthy nibbles can even help you get through a long commute with your appetite control intact.

Snacking Tips

Many people think that, when it comes to weight management, snacking is a no-no. But snacking can actually be good for you—if it's done right. Not only can it give you an opportunity to sneak extra nutrients into your daily dietary regimen, but it can also serve as a bridge from one meal to the next, which can help you avoid overeating. The key is to plan out your snacks ahead of time, rather than grabbing something spontaneously. The best snacks contain plenty of vitamins, minerals, fiber, and/or phytochemicals, and they consist of a reasonable portion. In other words, they should be measured out and eaten from a bowl or a dish, not from a box or bag. The following snacks can be consumed alone or in combination. *Bon appetit!*

- Fresh fruit, alone or dipped in nonfat yogurt or with unsalted peanut butter or low-fat string cheese
- Brown rice cakes spread with nut butter
- Cut fresh vegetables (baby carrots, celery, snap peas, bell peppers, cucumbers, tomatoes, zucchini) with salsa, hummus, or a nonfat bean dip
- Whole-grain pretzels or low-salt crackers

(continued)

- Dry whole-grain cereal
- A dried fruit and nut bar (e.g., a KIND bar) or a low-fat, low-sugar granola bar (Kashi makes good ones)
- Nuts and seeds without added oil or salt
- Air-popped popcorn
- Low-fat or nonfat yogurt by itself or with muesli
- Baked corn chips and salsa
- Low-fat cottage cheese and fruit
- A hardboiled egg

If you find it tempting to join in when you see others eating junk food at work, remove yourself from the workplace during mealtimes. Bring a healthy lunch and leave the office for a brisk walk, then eat your thoughtfully prepared food outside or in your car while listening to relaxing music. Time away may be just what the doctor ordered!

The Skill: Developing a Personal Food Policy for Eating Out

If you know you'll be going out to dinner, eat a light lunch; if you had a big lunch at a restaurant, consume a light, vegetable-dominant dinner at home. At the restaurant, consider asking your server to remove the bread or chip basket from the table so that you won't reach for the contents automatically and overeat before your meal arrives. Stick with water, club soda, unsweetened (iced or hot) tea, or another beverage without added sugar. Be careful about alcohol. For one thing, it provides quite a lot of calories. For another, it may disinhibit you, and without that restraint, you may eat far more than you otherwise would. If you do choose an alcoholic beverage, don't start drinking until after you start eating; sip slowly and savor; and alternate sips of your preferred alcoholic libation with sips of water to reduce the dose but not the pleasure.

Starting with a salad or a broth-based soup will help take the edge off your appetite. When possible, choose main dishes that include lots of vegetables, such as stir-fries, kabobs, or pasta primavera (with a tomato, rather than a cream, sauce). If the entrée portions are large, consider sharing one with a dining companion or make your entrée work double time by taking half of it home for tomorrow's lunch or dinner. Some people have the waiter divide the portion before it even reaches the table. In a 2007 survey of three hundred chefs, researchers from Clemson University investigated who is primarily responsible for determining portion sizes at restaurants and what factors go into the decision. Not surprisingly, presentation of the foods, cost issues, and customer expectations were the primary drivers of portion size. What was eye-opening? While 76 percent of the chefs surveyed believed they served "regular" portions, the actual servings of steak and pasta they were putting on the plates were two to four times larger than the U.S. government's recommended serving sizes. So before you lift a single forkful to your mouth, take a good look and see if yours is a reasonably sized portion. (You can use the guidelines in chapter 4 as a reality check.)

Stick with desserts that are primarily fresh fruit (as long as it's not covered with crème fraîche), fruit compotes or cobblers, or sorbets. Reserve decadent desserts for special occasions or for times when you can share with your tablemates. These are all decisions you can make ahead of time, before you even sit down at the table.

Occasionally, it's fine to vary your food policy. But for the sake of your efforts to establish healthier eating habits, try to stick to it as much as you can. That way, you'll be able to eat out without feeling diner's remorse the next day. Dining out will be the liberating, enjoyable experience it should be, before, during, and after the meal.

The Skill: Decoding Restaurant Menus

Dining at restaurants means you need to be your own food sleuth. As a starting point, read the menu carefully. You can automatically rule out

The Kid Factor

When dining out with kids, there's no rule that says you have to cater to them. You can choose restaurants that appeal to you *and* your kids. Look for those that offer healthy children's menus—basically smaller portions of adult meals, not just fried fare—and/or are willing to prepare plainer versions of adult foods (such as baked chicken, grilled seafood or meat, or pasta), perhaps with sauce on the side. You might choose two or three healthy options you know your child will like, then let your child pick from the narrowed-down list. When ordering from a kids' menu, substitute healthier sides such as carrots, green beans, or apple slices in place of fries whenever possible, and have your kids order skim milk or water to drink. In the meantime, you can seize the occasion as a "teachable moment" and take steps toward broadening your child's palate by offering a bite or two from whatever you order. You never know—your child might just have a hidden penchant for Arctic char!

anything described as "crusted" or "crispy," which usually means fried or even deep-fried. The same holds true of fare that's sautéed, since restaurants typically use more oil or butter than you'd use at home. Also, watch out for dishes that are described with words such as *buttered, creamed, battered, breaded, rich, smothered,* or *au gratin,* as all these words are a red flag for extra fat, cream, cheese—and calories.

In general, you're better off ordering something baked, broiled, grilled, poached, roasted, or steamed. When ordering meat, select leaner cuts such as round steak, filet mignon, or center-cut pork or lamb chops, and ask to have the skin removed from poultry before it's cooked. Look for freshly made entrée salads that offer a balanced meal in one dish—a variety of greens topped with chopped veggies; bits of egg, chicken, or seafood; and perhaps some nuts. You can also ask for low-fat dressing on the side, and skip the croutons.

Of course, menus that indicate nutritious or "heart-healthy" choices take the guesswork out of the ordering process. The same is true if the menu indicates the calorie content of the dishes. (Most fast-food chains have nutrition information; if it's not posted, you just need to ask for it.) In fact, researchers at Yale University found that when people were presented with menus that had calorie counts, they ordered items with fewer calories and consumed fewer calories during the meal than those who received the same menu without the calorie info; this effect is enhanced when the menus also mention the recommended daily calorie intake for adults. The trouble with just cutting calories is that you may be left hungry and eat more later. But if you trade up the overall nutritional quality of your choices, they will help give you a lasting feeling of fullness on fewer calories.

The Skill: Questioning Your Server and Making Healthy Requests

Often we're enticed simply by the language on a menu. After all, savvy chefs and menu designers know the seductive power of the artfully chosen adjective. They know that if they feed us the right descriptions, we'll throw caution to the wind and order that succulent potpie or that braised free-range chicken with crispy eggplant fritters. But it's a mistake to take menu offerings at face value, because some choices are deceptive. "Pan-seared Alaskan halibut" may sound as if it's lower in fat than a "grilled pork loin chop," but it depends on how much oil is added in the searing process. A pasta sauce that contains a dash of cream may sound like Diet Enemy Number One, but not if the chef put three tablespoons in a pot that could serve twelve.

The truth is that there's just no way to know what has been put in the food unless you've stood in the kitchen and watched the chef prepare it. Even experts have a hard time estimating fat and calorie content at restaurants. In a survey conducted by the Center for Science in the Public

Interest (CSPI) and researchers at New York University, professionally trained dietitians underestimated the fat content of five restaurant meals by an average of 49 percent, and misjudged the calorie content by an average of 37 percent.

That's why it's essential to ask your server specific questions about how a dish is prepared and what it contains. Don't assume anything. I have been surprised innumerable times by ingredients in restaurant dishes that have no business being there. The description on the menu may make no mention whatsoever of butter or cream, even when many other ingredients in the dish are listed. But I don't want to consume unhealthy, and unnecessary, butter or cream, so I've made it a routine to say, "I would like that with no butter or cream, please," even when I don't think it's in there. Usually it is!

Don't be shy about making requests; just try to keep them simple and reasonable. For example, you might ask for a baked potato or mixed greens in place of French fries, or to hold the mayonnaise on your sandwich. If a dish comes with bacon or sausage (both of which are notoriously high in fat), ask if you can substitute Canadian bacon or ham (both of which are lower in fat). Ask for dry toast at breakfast or brunch, since many kitchens butter it before serving it. Request sauce, gravy, or salad dressing on the side, and dip your fork into it before picking up a bite of food (rather than slathering it on the food). This will give you the flavor with every bite, but much less fat. If your entrée comes on a plate that's swimming with butter after you've requested no added fat, send it back. Most restaurants will alter their preparation methods if a customer requests it; if they won't, you should take your personal preferences to another restaurant that will! Sometimes it even pays to ask for larger portions of the side dishes, such as steamed or roasted veggies, and a smaller portion of the meat, poultry, or fish. Many restaurants will oblige, as this will actually save *them* money.

The Healthiest Orders by Cuisine

Italian

Choose minestrone, salads, pasta, grilled calamari or chicken, fish, seafood, or poultry dishes that have tomato-, olive oil–, or wine-based sauces. Steer clear of cream sauces, cheese- or meat-filled pastas, and dishes with excessive amounts of butter or cheese.

Chinese

Go with broth-based soups (think egg drop or hot and sour soup) and vegetarian, tofu, seafood, and poultry dishes that have lots of veggies. Avoid battered or deep-fried dishes and fried rice. Request minimal use of oil, and go with brown rice (instead of white) whenever possible.

Mexican

Choose grilled instead of fried chicken, fish, or meat dishes; and soft flour or corn tortillas rather than hard taco shells. Ask for black beans instead of refried beans, and avoid excessive amounts of cheese, sour cream, and tortilla chips from the bottomless basket; choose guacamole, which is healthy but high in calories, as a condiment in moderation.

French

Select salads; broth-based fish stews; steamed mussels; roasted chicken, meat, or fish; ratatouille; and dishes cooked in wine-based sauces. Watch out for excessive cream, butter, or cheese—and the nearly ubiquitous *frites* (a.k.a. French fries).

Japanese

Opt for broth-based or miso soups, edamame, salads, noodle soups, sushi or sashimi (with low-sodium soy sauce or rice wine

(continued)

vinegar), broiled meats, chicken, or seafood. Avoid tempura—even if it's vegetables or seafood; it's not a healthy choice.

Delis

Stick with whole-grain breads and lean cold cuts such as sliced turkey or chicken breast—instead of highly processed, fatty meats such as pastrami and corned beef—and load up with lettuce, tomato, and/or grilled veggies. Ask for mustard instead of mayo or butter.

Grills, diners, and fast-food joints

You can't go wrong with salads, as long as you avoid cheese, croutons, bacon bits, and mayonnaise-based potato or pasta salads. Request low-fat dressing on the side and use it sparingly. Avoid burgers and fried foods.

The Skill: Maintaining Control of Your Eating and Drinking While Socializing

The people who are sitting at a table with us can have overt or subtle influences on our eating patterns, often without our realizing it. In one study, researchers from the Netherlands manipulated portion sizes and the food intake of others during a twenty-minute eating occasion to see what effect this would have. As it turned out, the participants consumed more when they were offered a larger portion, and they ate more when their companion ate more—a potentially harmful double whammy! In a separate study, these same researchers found that women were more likely to take a bite of their meal within five seconds of their dining companion than to eat at their own pace—a powerful example of what's known as "behavioral mimicry."

And yet we're usually unaware of these dynamics. In two studies published in *Health Psychology*, researchers paired up 122 women to examine how the presence and behavior of a dining companion would influence the amount of food the other person consumed in an eating setting. In both studies, there were strong similarities between the amounts of food each member of each pair consumed, but most participants identified hunger and taste as the primary drivers of their intake, not their partner's behavior. This is called the "social facilitation" effect, and it essentially means that the sheer presence of other people at the table is likely to make you eat and drink more than if you were dining alone.

In the real world, when you're sharing a meal with others during a holiday get-together, a dinner party, or even a restaurant gathering, it's easy to lose sight of how much, or even what, you're consuming. Your hand may pass back and forth to the bread plate or tortilla chip basket more times than you'd care to count. You may reach for seconds (or thirds) if the serving bowl is near you, just because of the sheer proximity of it. Perhaps this is partly because when you're with company you enjoy, you relax, which also can cause you to loosen the reins of your dietary restraint. Plus, dining with others means sitting at the table longer, which can make you continue to pick at food that's on the table even if you've had enough.

It's also easy for your dietary resolve to become derailed when you're at a party or social event where the unspoken mantra seems to be "eat, drink, and be merry." Fortunately, it is possible to have a good time without overeating or regretting your dietary actions the next day—if you get into the right mind-set ahead of time. It helps if you reinforce your sense of competence and confidence before you go to the social event. If you tell yourself, "I'm a strong, healthy person and I plan to stay that way," in the hours leading up to the event, you'll walk into the party feeling empowered to stick with your healthy approach to eating. Exercising before the event can also make a difference: Besides burning calories ahead of time, physical activity can make you more responsive to your body's hunger and satiety cues and help you organize your eating behavior better while you're socializing. Exercise also relieves stress and anxiety, so if you're susceptible to social jitters, a workout can help you arrive at the scene with a clear head and be less prone to eating for emotional reasons.

It may sound counterintuitive, but eating something, preferably with protein (perhaps a hardboiled egg or a piece of cheese and an apple), and drinking some water beforehand can help take the edge off your hunger and fortify your resolve when you arrive. Once you're there, start with lower-calorie foods (vegetables or a broth-based soup, for example) so you have better control with other items. You could also offer to bring a dish to the party—and make it a beautiful platter of crudités with a low-fat dip or a colorful fruit salad. That way, you'll know there will be at least one item that's healthy and low in calories, something you know you can indulge in freely. (Since most adults in the United States struggle with their weight, others at the gathering may welcome a healthy option.) And the hosts will appreciate your contribution because it means one less dish for them to plan and prepare.

From the *Things-You-Never-Knew-You-Never-Knew* Files

People who are overweight tend to eat larger meals away from home than people whose weight is normal, according to research at Sam Houston State University in Texas. The theory: Overweight people seem to be more susceptible to appetite-stimulating environmental cues. Another body of research suggests that people eat more when other people are overeating.

Consciously eat slowly, chewing your food thoroughly, and pause periodically to gauge how satisfied you are. Make an effort to eat more slowly than everyone else at the table or gathering. If you're the last person to start eating and the last one to finish, you'll enjoy the food more (by savoring the flavors) and you'll be satisfied with less (and less likely to take second helpings). Given your timing, your hosts may not even notice how much you are (or aren't) eating.

At any social event, it helps if you remind yourself that the real reason you're there is to see people you know and perhaps meet some new ones; the food really is secondary. Staying mindful of this helps curb the impulsive eating that can be easy to do at parties. It also helps to remove the focus from food altogether by identifying specific people you want to meet or talk to. That way, you can have a good time, regardless of what you do or don't eat.

The Skill: Standing Up to Food Pushers

At first blush, this may seem surprising, but peer pressure with food is actually quite common—and yet a bit mystifying. After all, you don't just get into any car and drive it; presumably you drive only your own car. You probably don't routinely use a coworker's lipstick or handkerchief. And you probably don't let anyone else decide what you will wear on a given day, whether you will take an umbrella, or whether you will use perfume or deodorant. So the idea that someone else would make food-related decisions for us is just plain odd. But somehow we find it acceptable to let other people decide what, when, and how much we eat.

Since time immemorial, human beings have shown each other love and affection with treats, foods, and feasts. Parents love their children with French fries, lollipops, and ice cream. Mothers and grandmothers from many different cultural backgrounds often lavish love in the form of copious servings of food—with a side dish of guilt if you complain about eating it all. *There are starving kids in China, you know!* (In fact, there are, but overall, China is succumbing to the global obesity epidemic as it modernizes.) Meanwhile, at family gatherings, office lunches, or other social events, people may encourage you to eat more than you're inclined to and/or more than you should. Often it's because that's what they're doing, and they want you to join them.

One solution is to try to raise the bar. Instead of succumbing to peer pressure, tell people about your resolve to eat more healthfully and ask them to support you in your efforts. Remember: The majority of adults in the United States is overweight and many are dealing with a chronic health problem (such as hypertension or diabetes) that's related to those excess pounds, so you may have a positive influence on those in your social circle. Instead of letting other people undermine your resolve, inspire them to join you in your quest for better nutrition and better health and to enlist valuable support from one another. There's no rule that says only *unhealthy* eating habits can be contagious, so why not spread your healthy dietary approach to friends and loved ones?

If this tactic doesn't work, you can always shift gears and go to plan B: Set firm limits when people push rich dishes or second helpings by explaining that you're making an effort to eat more lightly so you can lose weight, reduce your cholesterol, or lower your blood pressure, for example. That way, you won't say anything negative about what they're eating or offering but you can stand your ground on health reasons. Sometimes people are more willing to accept a health-related reason for changing your eating patterns than a weight-related one. Somehow it seems less open to negotiation.

If you feel obligated to have the cake or whatever is being served because the host went to a lot of trouble or the occasion is a big deal, you can give the impression that you're indulging: Eat one or two bites so it looks like you're joining in, then push your plate aside. Or you could say it looks fabulous but you can't eat another bite of anything after the delicious meal you just enjoyed, and ask if you could take home a piece for the next day. At that point, whether you eat it or give it away will be your decision, no pressure.

The Skill: Sidestepping Sabotage or Turning It into Support

Even among close friends or family members, you may encounter sabotage or *social undermining*, as it's called in the research literature. It can go something like this: You're trying to slim down, but maybe your friends push you to have another slice of pizza or your significant other brings you a box of chocolates to cheer you up—the very stuff you're trying to avoid! Sometimes the sabotage is well meaning—people who care about you may see you struggling and just want you to feel better—and sometimes it isn't.

Often it's more about the saboteur than it is about you. The person may feel threatened by your efforts to lose weight or feel worried that a change in your health, vitality, or appearance will change the dynamic in the relationship (in which case, a little reassurance about how much you care for him or her may be in order). The person may envy your ability to take charge of your health and may feel inferior by comparison. Sometimes people just resist change—even if it's *you* who's making the change—because they're comfortable with the status quo. And sometimes sabotage reflects outdated ways of showing love—by providing bountiful food, instead of verbal (or other) expressions of love and affection.

Ultimately, it doesn't matter if the sabotage is conscious or unconscious, well intentioned or malicious. In the end, it's up to you to handle it. Let's start with the ugly kind, because that's simpler to dispose of. If sabotage is coming from someone who genuinely seems to want you to fail in achieving your goals, avoid, ignore, or chastise that person as you see fit.

On the other hand, if the sabotage is unconscious and/or well intentioned, and it's coming from a friend or loved one, calmly talk to the person about it and explain that you need his help and what form of help would be most welcome. You might say something like "As you know, I'm trying to lose weight (or eat more healthfully), and I know your intentions are good when you offer me dessert (or whatever it is), but I'd actually appreciate it if you didn't, because it's hard to resist temptation! What I'd really appreciate is your help and support to keep me on track. Can I count on you for that?" Sabotage works only in the shadows, so once you point it out, it's likely to wither and die.

Even better, you'll be replacing a problem with a new solution: *social contracting*. Entering into an agreement with someone you care about is a highly effective way to modify your behavior. For one thing, when you ask someone to help you, you're making your goals public, which helps you stay accountable. For another, you now have another form of social support because you're engaging that person in the process of changing your lifestyle. Just be sure to be as specific as possible in telling that person how she can best help you, whether it's with a well-timed pep talk, helping to monitor your behavior, or joining you in your quest for healthier eating. Take the guesswork out of the picture.

There's no need to choose between spending time with others and eating healthfully. With some effort, you can turn dangerous liaisons into valuable sources of support that will help you reach your goals for improving your diet and your health. Think of it as a way to turn the tables from potentially negative influences on your eating habits to positive, health-promoting ones.

THE DISEASE-PROOF TO-DO LIST:

- Plan ahead and take charge of your eating habits at work by bringing your own meals and snacks.
- Develop a personal food policy for dining out by deciding what and how much you'll eat and drink—and stick with it.
- Identify kid-friendly, healthy restaurants (or menu options), offering healthy foods that are served in child-appropriate servings.
- Stick with reasonable-size portions and take the rest home—or share a meal.
- Learn how to decipher restaurant menus by looking for key words.
- Ask your server the right questions about ingredients and preparation techniques, and request smart, healthy substitutions or omissions.
- Take steps (such as having a snack before you go and focusing on socializing, not eating) to control your food and beverage intake at social events.
- Politely confront, elude, or defy food pushers; don't give in to them just to make them happy.
- Give the slip to sabotage and/or try to turn saboteurs into allies by asking for their help in specific ways.

Ten

Move Your Body, Lose the Health Risks

The Challenge: Technological advances have replaced old-fashioned muscle power. Thanks to this and our modern hectic schedules, regular physical activity is hard to get.

The Right Response: Recognize physical activity as the priority it deserves to be, and a natural state to which our bodies are designed and adapted. Physical activity, like sleep, pays dividends on the time invested in it, by enhancing health, concentration, motivation, and overall productivity.

The Relevant Skills: Appreciating the benefits of regular physical activity; discovering your personal motivation for becoming more active; challenging your excuses for not exercising; finding physical activities that suit your style; framing an exercise program properly; making time for workouts; keeping your workouts fresh and inspiring; and learning to love the vitality of being physically active.

A sedentary lifestyle is a major risk factor for heart disease, stroke, diabetes, osteoporosis, many forms of cancer, and premature death. Conversely, regular physical activity has been shown to reduce the risks of developing cardiovascular disease, type 2 diabetes, hypertension, breast and colon cancer, and many other life-threatening diseases. Compared to being sedentary, routine physical activity can cut the risk of developing any major chronic disease in half. That's right—*in half!*

Physical inactivity has long been recognized as one of the top three causes of premature death in the United States, but a recent review of the global evidence, published in *The Lancet*, indicates that physical inactivity is now responsible for nearly 10 percent of the world's annual mortality. Moreover, in a study involving 222,497 people ages forty-five and older, researchers at the University of Sydney in Australia found that the risk of dying from any cause was 15 percent higher among those who sit for eight to ten hours a day and 40 percent higher among those who sit for eleven hours a day or longer. The pattern was consistent among men and women, overweight people and thin folks, and people who exercise as well as those who don't. In other words, spending many hours a day sitting is simply harmful to your health, even if you are physically active when you're not resting on your tush.

From an evolutionary perspective, human beings were built for movement, not spending long hours sitting on our derrieres. In this age of automated everything, we have essentially engineered movement right out of our lives. We no longer hunt or gather; we order takeout food, often for delivery. We do our banking online and use direct deposit. We no longer have to walk to a colleague's office to confer on a matter; phone or e-mail is the go-to mode of communication. We no longer have to go shopping for groceries, clothes, furniture, or other items; we can order what we want or need on our computers and have it sent directly to our homes.

Exercise has been squeezed out of the average day for both adults and kids. Despite the epidemics of obesity and type 2 diabetes in children, more and more schools are cutting back on physical education programs, rather than expanding them. This is happening even though there's solid evidence that good physical activity programs during the school day preserve or enhance academic performance, rather than interfering with it. According to a study by researchers at the University of Tennessee, Knoxville, middle-school students who are more physically fit (especially on measures of cardiorespiratory endurance, muscular strength, and stamina) achieve better grades and perform better than their classmates on standardized tests. For years, approximately 40 percent of adults in the United States reported that they never exercise. More recent studies are painting an even worse picture: Using accelerometers to measure actual movement, instead of relying on study participants' self-reports, the latest research indicates that only 3.5 percent of adults in the United States between the ages of eighteen and fifty-nine achieve the minimum amount of physical activity that's recommended by the government: 150 minutes of moderate-intensity activity per week. *Only 3.5 percent!*

This lifestyle has given rise to a phenomenon now being referred to in research circles as "sedentarism," which is variously described as expending less than 10 percent of your daily energy (or calories) performing moderate to vigorous physical activities, spending an inordinate amount of time sitting down during your leisure time, or a combination of the two. In popular culture, by contrast, *sedentarism* usually refers to extended engagement in behaviors that involve little movement and low calorie expenditure (such as watching TV). Meanwhile, "sedentary physiology"—the opposite of "exercise physiology"—has become an increasingly rich area of scientific inquiry, because this behavior has such serious, deleterious health consequences. Any way you look at it, we are gaining weight and increasing our risks of chronic diseases by the seat of our pants, not the soles of our shoes.

It shouldn't be this way. Fortunately, the solution is fairly simple: *Move more! Really!* A 2012 study published in the *British Medical Journal* suggests a potential gain in life expectancy of two years, on average, just from reducing total daily sitting to less than three hours. (Admittedly, this is hard for office workers to do, but even getting up and moving more often throughout the day will help.) As little as twenty minutes of aerobic exercise five times a week can be the difference between an at-risk child developing type 2 diabetes or not, according to a study reported in *JAMA*. We know from the Diabetes Prevention Program that modest improvements in weight, activity, and diet can prevent diabetes in nearly two out of three at-risk adults. The largest available database on sustained weight loss, the National Weight Control Registry, shows that even moderate daily activity appears to be a nearly universal element in helping people who've lost substantial amounts of weight successfully maintain that loss over the long term. And research from the University of Colorado, Boulder, has found that while healthy older adults tend to experience increased expression of several genes that promote inflammation and oxidative stress, regular habitual exercise ameliorates these effects.

The Skill: Appreciating the Benefits of Regular Physical Activity

In recent years there has been a steady, resonant drumbeat of news rapping out the profound health benefits of even modest levels of physical activity. And there's no mystery as to why: During physical activity, there's more oxygen in your blood, increased blood flow to your muscles and lungs, and the release of natural painkillers (such as endorphins), which boost your sense of well-being. Regular exercise produces numerous physiological benefits, including controlling blood pressure, cholesterol, and blood sugar; and it reduces hidden harmful inflammation in the body, which can lower your risk of developing a variety of chronic diseases.

Over time, regular aerobic exercise also leads to increased stamina, better weight control, a stronger heart, a boost in mood, stronger muscles, and enhanced immune function, potentially helping to prevent infectious diseases such as cold and flu as well as long-term threats such as cancer. Weight-bearing exercise and strength-training workouts build and protect your bone mass, thereby reducing your risk of developing osteoporosis. And exercise improves sexual function, in both women and men, by balancing hormones and enhancing blood flow to sexual organs (thus heightening sexual function and responsiveness) and by boosting a person's self-image, which is also important for getting in the mood. Recent research from New Zealand even found that exercise helps reduce cravings and withdrawal symptoms while people are quitting smoking.

But that's not all. Regular exercise can also reduce the risk of recurrence of a variety of diseases. That's why cardiac rehab programs—which are designed to help people recover from heart attacks and heart surgery—include physical activity to help strengthen the heart and blood vessels and help prevent another cardiac event. Moreover, after reviewing the medical literature, researchers at the National Cancer Institute found "consistent evidence" that among cancer survivors physical activity is even associated with reduced mortality from breast cancer, colon cancer, and other causes.

The Fitness vs. Fatness Debate

Many studies show that independent of body weight, a person's fitness level has major implications for her health and vitality, chronic disease risk, and even life span. Dr. Steven Blair of the Cooper Clinic in Texas is famously associated with the "fatness versus fitness" debate, pointing out that one can be fit even if heavy, and that the health benefits of fitness pertain just the same. Without question, there are advantages to being both lean and fit, and you can certainly use exercise to help you lose weight (if you boost the "calories out" part of the energy-balance equation while controlling the calories you consume). If you walk at a moderate pace for a half hour, you will burn a couple of hundred calories. Do that daily and keep your food intake constant, and you could lose a half a pound a week. Do it for a year, and that's 25 pounds of weight you could drop.

But that's not the real measure of how valuable exercise is. If you exercise muscles so they grow a bit—not so they're big and bulky but so they're lean and strong—you'll end up with more muscle mass. Lean muscle mass is more metabolically active than

(continued)

body fat is, which means it burns more fuel (or calories) even when you're resting. So if you add a pound of muscle mass to your body, you will burn 30 to 50 more calories a day on average just to maintain your current weight. Exercise, say, twenty minutes three times a week, in other words, and you will burn more calories while you sleep! Talk about a strong return on your investment.

The bottom line: Physical fitness is good for each and every one of us, whatever our size or shape may be. What's more, regular exercise has been found to play a crucial role in helping people who've lost considerable amounts of weight maintain their leaner status. In the National Weight Control Registry, the best database we have for successful long-term maintenance of significant weight loss, routine physical activity is almost universally part of the winning formula.

If all this isn't enough to get you off the couch, consider this: Exercise is good for our brain function and our emotional state of mind. It enhances blood and oxygen delivery to the brain (as well as the body), reducing the risk of Alzheimer's and other forms of dementia, while improving concentration and productivity. (In fact, new research published in the *Annals of Internal Medicine* found that people who have the highest levels of cardiorespiratory fitness at midlife are 36 percent less likely to be diagnosed with dementia in later life.)

Exercise also sets the stage for learning, memory, and recall. It enhances mood and attention and eases anxiety and depression. In fact, research at Duke University has found that aerobic exercise is as effective as antidepressants in treating major depression—but people who rely on movement therapy have lower relapse rates than those taking meds do. Exercise also mitigates some of the effects of stress and even reverses certain aspects of aging in the brain. These effects may be partly due to the exercise-induced release of mood-boosting endorphins; other neurotransmitters (brain chemicals) such as serotonin, norepinephrine, and dopamine; and brain-derived neurotrophic factor (BDNF).

Yet, as John Ratey, MD, notes in *Spark: The Revolutionary New Science of Exercise and the Brain*, even many psychiatrists don't recognize that stress overload can erode the vital connections between nerve cells in the brain or that chronic depression can actually shrink certain areas of the brain. "And they don't know that, conversely, exercise unleashes a cascade of neurochemicals and growth factors that can reverse this process, physically bolstering the brain's infrastructure," he notes. "In fact, the brain responds like muscles do, growing with use, withering with inactivity."

There's no disputing that physical activity is good for our bodies and minds, and yet the vast majority of us get too little of it. The fact is, we all have a native animal vitality inside us, one that should be respected, honored, and nurtured. It's the opposite of disability. Think about it: When you see someone in a wheelchair, you might feel sorry for him because his freedom of movement is restricted. Yet those of us who are fortunate to have healthy legs often neglect to make use of them; we're squandering our own physical abilities. If you think about it that way, you might see that we are engaging in a subtle but common form of cognitive dissonance. Our feet were made for walking and running, dancing and skipping, jumping and climbing. The vitality that comes from physical activity and good health makes life more enjoyable and can't be replicated with any technological advance. Why would any of us voluntarily throw this away? If someone tried to take it from us by force, we would surely fight to defend it! Objectively speaking, making a case for routine physical activity is a cinch, and the evidence could scarcely be any stronger. Move your body every day, and you'll add years to your life, and better quality to those years. Just sit on it, and you will very likely lose both. It's a simple choice, really.

The Skill: Discovering Your Personal Motivation for Becoming More Active

Understanding and valuing all the potential physiological and psychological benefits that stem from regular exercise will help motivate you to embrace physical activity as something you *want* to do, instead of viewing it as something you simply *should* do. But you might need to nudge your motivation in the right direction. As previously noted, it's common for people to have conflicting motivations in life. Maybe you do want to exercise more (perhaps to reap the health benefits) but have reasons you *don't* want to (perhaps because of time constraints)—these conflicting rationales can lead to ambivalence about changing your habits. Fortunately, you can tilt the scale in a positive direction by taking stock of all the pros and cons of increasing your level of physical activity versus remaining sedentary.

One of the easiest ways to do this is by creating a decision-balance chart (described in chapter 2), in which you list all the anticipated advantages of making a change in one column and the disadvantages of doing so in an adjacent column. You can keep it this simple or you can expand the chart to include the advantages of not making a change along with the disadvantages of that particular choice (see Table 5.1). If you can then find new items to add to the "Advantages" column under "Increasing Physical Activity" or the "Disadvantages" under "Remaining Sedentary," or, if you can think of reasons to remove some of the disadvantages of increasing physical activity or the advantages of remaining sedentary, your analysis will lead to a new conclusion. If the pros don't naturally outweigh the cons on your list, you can challenge your reasons for not changing so that you tilt the balance in favor of making the change.

You might intentionally stack the deck in favor of physical activity by noting all the benefits to your body, mind, and waistline that can come from exercising regularly—improved cardiovascular, respiratory, and immune function; more energy and an enhanced sense of well-being; less anxiety and depression and better mood regulation; greater muscle tone and definition; an improved complexion; better sex; and so on. It may take some active thinking to generate sufficient enthusiasm for changing your behavior, but it's worth the effort. Ideally, some of the information just given will help, but only you can decide when you are ready. It's your ambivalence—only you can change it.

Table 5.1. A Decision Balance Chart for Increasing Physical Activity

Increasing Physical Activity			
ADVANTAGES	It could help me lose weight.	**DISADVANTAGES**	It's hard work.
	I'll protect my health and brain.		It takes time.
	I'll have more energy.		I hate Spandex.
	I'll improve my sex life.		My joints hurt when I exercise.
	My moods will take a turn for the better.		
Remaining Sedentary			
ADVANTAGES	It's easy.	**DISADVANTAGES**	This won't help me lose weight.
	I'll save time.		This won't improve my health.
	I won't have to sweat.		I could gain weight.
	I won't be in any discomfort.		I won't feel more vibrant.
			I won't gain muscle definition.

Simply by constructing the decision balance chart and reviewing it, you may find that the motivation you need to move forward increases naturally. The more personal you can make the reasons in favor of taking the plunge, the better. The truth is, we talk ourselves into things every day; think of this as an opportunity to convince yourself that it's worth doing something that's good for your body, mind, and lifespan. Keep a copy of this chart accessible so that you can consult it if or when your motivation to head to the gym, jogging trail, or court wanes. Another important consideration: Maybe you are motivated to exercise but are just too intimidated to start. You know how worthwhile it is, but it just seems too hard, you don't know how to make the time, and so on. If that's the case, then read on, because much of this chapter (and the following one) is about making it easier.

From the *Things-You-Never-Knew-You-Never-Knew* Files

Recently, a study from the Netherlands found that exposure to exercise commercials had an interesting effect: Those who watched exercise-related commercials before eating lunch consumed approximately 22 percent fewer calories in the meal than those who watched neutral commercials. The implication? Keeping fitness-related messages in mind can help you keep your eating habits under control.

The Skill: Challenging Your Excuses for Not Exercising

Many people are experts when it comes to coming up with reasons for why they can't exercise. Few of these excuses are valid. In fact, exercise is important enough to so many aspects of what makes life good that it should be a priority for us all. Over the years, I've heard from patients that they are too busy to find time for exercise; I've always been inclined to think I was too busy *not to*, because the benefits far outweigh the costs in time expended.

When investigating the most common barriers people encounter with physical activity, my research team at Yale found that lack of knowledge about how to begin an exercise regimen, time and scheduling challenges, lack of social support, insufficient motivation or energy, and financial limitations were at the top of the list. The good news is: there are skills and strategies that can help the vast majority of people climb over or go around these barriers and become more physically active. Let's take these obstacles to exercise in reverse order. Financial limitations are the easiest barrier to dispense with because you can go for a walk or run for free. It doesn't cost you a cent! Much the same is true about turning on the radio and dancing for half an hour. Wherever you live, there is almost certainly an inexpensive, if not downright free, way to get some motion into your day.

As far as insufficient motivation and energy go, motivation is something you may have to work on, as previously noted, but the energy issue is easier to deal with. As surprising as it may be, scientific evidence has increasingly suggested that regular exercise can combat feelings of low energy and fatigue in healthy adults. Besides building strength and stamina, aerobic exercise boosts the flow of blood and oxygen throughout your body and mind, making you feel more alert, more focused, and more energetic. Often exercise has an invigorating effect, but if you find that you don't feel recharged after you exercise, try exercising at different times of day or at different intensities until you find the one that rejuvenates you. (If your energy shortage is the result of poor sleep, see chapter 12.) Meanwhile, there are many ways to deal with the issue of social support (or lack thereof), whether it's by joining a gym with a friend, finding a workout buddy, or swapping childcare duties with your spouse or a neighbor so you can each find time to exercise.

The point is, with some creative thinking, you should be able to challenge and refute your excuses one by one. Listen to the things you claim are holding you back from exercising, then consider, first, whether what you're claiming is actually true; and second, how you can get around the obstacle or find a way to deal with it effectively. It also helps to give yourself reminders about all the different ways you stand to benefit from regular physical activity, which will fortify your resolve to find ways around those obstacles.

While many people believe that only vigorous, continuous exercise will yield health benefits, that's simply not true. Accumulating twenty to thirty minutes of physical activity over the course of a day—even if it's by doing such routine things as taking the stairs or walking around a shopping mall—can confer as much as 85 percent of the cardiovascular benefits of vigorous exercise. Interestingly, a study at Arizona State University, in Phoenix, found that when men with prehypertension (a precursor to high blood pressure) did three ten-minute sessions of aerobic exercise spread out evenly throughout the day, they experienced greater declines in their systolic blood pressure over twenty-four hours than those who did one continuous thirty-minute exercise session. So short bouts of exercise really do add up to health benefits!

The Skill: Finding Physical Activities That Suit Your Style

The key is to identify activities that suit your personal preferences and lifestyle, and to choose forms of movement that comfort you (the exercise equivalent of comfort food), energize you, or bring you pleasure in some way. For physical activity to have staying power, you have to enjoy it and get other benefits besides just the physical ones. What's right for you, in this respect, may be quite different from what's best for a friend, colleague, or neighbor. If you like to run, run. If you like to hike, hike. If you like to dance, dance. Don't assume that you don't like to exercise just because you don't like some particular form of exercise. Your body was made to move, but what moves you toward physical activity is unique to you.

When choosing physical activities that are likely to be a good fit for you, consider what you really want to get out of exercise physically, psychologically, emotionally, and socially. Do you have lots of energy, a competitive streak, or a side that seeks an adrenaline rush? What degree of thinking, strategizing, and other forms of mental engagement do you prefer to have with physical activity? Or maybe you simply want to be able to loosen up your stiff muscles and release pent-up energy after hours spent sitting at a desk. Maybe you want to release frustration and stress when you feel overwhelmed. Maybe your priority is to engage in a mind-body activity that makes you feel centered, anchored, and peaceful. Or maybe you want to have a sense of camaraderie and connection to other people as you move.

If you're entirely new to exercise, you may have to go through some trial and error by test-driving different activities to see which suit you or by asking friends and family members or even instructors at a gym what certain activities are really like and which might appeal to you. Once you've honestly assessed these elements, it's easier to match activities to your personal preferences. For example, if you value the social element, you might enjoy taking a class, joining a walking or cycling club, or walking or jogging with a friend; the added benefits are that you can help keep each other motivated and accountable. (It's harder to shirk a workout when someone is counting on you.) If you don't like to get breathless or too sweaty, you might prefer gentler group exercise, such as yoga or Pilates. For those who do enjoy pushing their limits, a Spinning class might be a great way to go. But if you prefer to fly solo, jogging, cycling, swimming, progressive weight training, or using cardio machines such as a stair-climber or elliptical machine on your own might suit you better.

From the *Things-You-Never-Knew-You-Never-Knew* Files

Research from Norway suggests that muscles retain a memory of their former fitness levels, even if they're currently withering from lack of use. After the nuclei in muscle cells proliferate in response to strength training (the form of exercise used in this study), those extra nuclei aren't lost during later periods of inactivity; they're actually retained in distinct muscle fibers. So just as you never forget how to ride a bike, your muscles actually remember how to lift weights, swing a racquet, or slalom on skis if you used to regularly engage in those activities—and they can regain their previous fitness level with retraining.

If you have a competitive nature, you might enjoy playing tennis, squash, or racquetball. If you prefer to collaborate, a team sport (such as basketball, volleyball, or soccer), mountain biking with a group, or even taking a highly synchronized dance class may be appealing to you. And if you like to concentrate and stay focused during physical activity, racquet sports or martial arts (such as tai chi or karate) might be good choices for you. By contrast, if zoning out or doing something rhythmic is more your style, using a cardio machine while listening to music may be the way to go; swimming or skating may appeal to you as well. There really is some form of physical activity that will appeal to every person.

The Skill: Framing an Exercise Program Properly

Some physical activity can be orchestrated into your day quite easily, just by choosing motion whenever the opportunity arises. Every little bit of movement counts. (The next chapter will address the stealth approach.) And exercise doesn't have to be done all at once. It can be, if that approach works for you, but it can also be accumulated over the course of the day. From a health-promoting standpoint, the goal is to get thirty minutes of moderate aerobic activity five days each week, and there are as many ways to get there as your imagination can conjure up.

A complete physical fitness program should include the elements of cardiorespiratory (a.k.a. aerobic) fitness, muscular strength and endurance, and flexibility. That may sound like a tall order, but it doesn't have to be if you use the FITT formula, which is recommended by most fitness organizations:

F is for frequency: This refers to how often you do a particular form of exercise. The recommendations call for five thirty-minute sessions of moderate-intensity aerobic activity per week; two to three nonconsecutive days each week of strength training; and stretching exercises to maintain flexibility at least two to three days per week.

I is for intensity: There are fancy numerical values you can use to determine the intensity of aerobic exercise, but my recommendation is to keep it simple. Moderately intense exercise means you're aware of an increase in your heart rate and breathing rate, but you can still speak in complete sentences. If it's difficult to talk, you've crossed the threshold from moderate to vigorous. The recommendations are for moderate-intensity aerobic activity most days of the week for a total of 150 minutes per week (minimum); if you opt for vigorous exercise, the recommended minimum is 75 minutes per week. As for strength training, you should do it to the point of muscle fatigue (not failure), while maintaining proper form; typically two to three sets of eight to twenty repetitions are advised. Stretching should be done to the point of mild tension, not discomfort.

T is for time: For aerobic activity, you can go for thirty to sixty minutes of continuous or intermittent activity (ten-minute bouts accumulated throughout the day); for strength training, twenty to sixty minutes is usually sufficient; for stretching, the goal is to hold each stretch for twenty to sixty seconds before moving on to the next one.

T is for type: Cardiorespiratory (or aerobic) activity is anything that's continuous and uses greater oxygen uptake and large muscle groups. This includes walking, jogging, cycling, swimming, stair-climbing, dancing, skating, skiing, using cardio machines, or playing movement-related sports (such as tennis or soccer). Strength-training activities challenge the musculoskeletal system with resistance in the form of weights, weight machines, resistance bands, kettlebells, or your own body weight. Flexibility exercises include anything that focuses on elongating the muscles and moving joints safely through their full range of motion (stretching, yoga, Pilates, and the like).

Choose whatever activities you like and mix and match them in any way that appeals to you. You can bundle physical activity as you like—all at once or spread out—every day or most days of the week. The important thing is to aim for the FITT targets, any way that works for you.

Exercise by the Numbers

If you want to develop a more physically active lifestyle, in addition to paying attention to the FITT formula, here are some other important numbers to keep in mind to help you exercise safely and consistently:

Ten minutes: If you don't feel like exercising on a given day, commit to doing just ten minutes of something—taking a brisk walk or riding a bike, for example. Chances are you'll feel better and decide to keep going. If you don't, at least you will have done something to boost your health and weight-control efforts.

Forty-eight hours: That's the maximum number of hours—two days!—that you should go without exercising if you're trying to make physical activity a habit.

10–20 percent: As you make progress in your fitness level, this is the most you should increase the intensity or duration of your workout from one week to the next—to prevent injuries or burnout. So if you've been walking briskly for thirty minutes a day for a while, it's best to increase the duration to thirty-three or thirty-six minutes for at least a week before trying to go longer.

Ten thousand: This is the current recommendation for how many steps you should try to take per day. Make tracking easier with an inexpensive pedometer.

The Skill: Making Time for Workouts

It's ideal if you can choose an activity and a venue that easily fit into your usual schedule. If you can find a gym, court, or jogging trail that's close to your home or workplace, it will be easier to slip in physical activity on a regular basis. (If you have young kids at home, you may want to choose a health club that offers childcare.) Try to carve out a dedicated time of day when there aren't likely to be conflicts with other aspects of your schedule—perhaps early in the morning, at your lunch break, or in the early evening. If you get in the habit of treating this time as sacred—you might even block out that time in your day planner as if it were an important business or doctor's appointment—you'll be more likely to stick with your exercise routine over time. This is how healthy habits are born!

When your calendar begins to get crowded, you can multitask in a positive way by making exercise social. Instead of meeting a friend or a colleague for drinks or dinner after work, take an evening exercise class or go for a brisk walk or jog together. Similarly, you can combine family time with exercise by going for a hike or bike ride or playing tag with your kids. Bringing people whose company you enjoy into the exercise equation will help keep physical activity lively, fresh, and inspiring, qualities that have a positively reinforcing effect on incorporating more movement in your life.

From the *Things-You-Never-Knew-You-Never-Knew* Files

Some research suggests that people are more likely to stick with an exercise program if they do it in the morning, presumably because unexpected challenges haven't had a chance to get in the way yet at the start of the day. Another benefit has emerged for being a morning mover and shaker. Research from Brigham Young University in Utah suggests that a moderate-to-vigorous bout of exercise in the morning may stave off cravings for the rest of the day.

The Skill: Keeping Your Workouts Fresh and Inspiring

As we all know, variety is the spice of life. It's what keeps things interesting, novel, and stimulating. Just as eating the same foods again and again can get boring, doing the same form of exercise or the same fitness routine every day can grow dull, too. (Admittedly, some people like the predictability and consistency of sticking with a particular exercise routine; if you're among them, there's no need to fix what isn't broken!) But if exercise monogamy is leading to exercise monotony, and it's starting to talk you out of moving and shaking, then it's time to shake up your routine.

There are several ways to do this. One is to cross-train—by doing different forms of movement on different days (walking one day, dancing or biking the next, swimming after that, and so on)—which provides the added benefits of challenging different muscles and preventing overuse injuries. Another option is to stick with your usual routine but to add an element of novelty—perhaps by inviting a friend to join you, making a new playlist, or doing it in a different setting.

It also helps to change up the intensity of a given routine by alternating bursts of faster walking or jogging with your regular pace. This approach is called *interval training*, and it can rev up your metabolism more than exercising at a comfortable, steady speed. Think of it as a way of tricking your body into burning calories faster. Cranking up the pace at intervals burns more calories during the workout; plus, upping the amount of energy (calories) burned during the workout means it will take your body longer to recover afterward. (You'll continue to burn more calories for a few hours after you've stopped exercising.)

You might notice that as you get fitter, your body will adapt to doing the same workout day after day. The good news is this means you've gotten fitter. The bad news is you won't burn as many calories for a given effort as you did initially. Regularly switching up the type of activity you do, along with the pace and intensity, will coax your body into burning calories faster both during the workout and afterward.

The Skill: Learning to Love the Vitality of Being Physically Active

My father, seventy-three (as I write this), is a cardiologist, and he's as fit as can be for predictable reasons: a lifetime of eating well and staying very active. It's something of a tradition for the two of us to go hiking in a nearby state park on Christmas Day. A few years ago we were doing just that on an especially crisp, cold, bright day. There had been a bit of early snow that season, and there was still some on the ground and in the trees. The late afternoon sun filtered through tree limbs, reflecting off icy surfaces. It was a stunningly beautiful scene.

At one point, after we had made our way up an incline that was moderately steep and fairly long, we were both breathing hard enough for the mist in our breath to form clouds of condensation in the air in front of us. So there we were with our frosty breath in the crisp air, the snow crunching beneath our feet, and the sun glinting off ice crystals, talking about the beauty of the woods and how great it felt to be doing what we were doing. Then the conversation took an interesting turn: We started talking about the innumerable patients we had each cared for over the years who could no longer enjoy something like this. Their health had declined too far—in many cases, because they had let it slip away—and they would never again have the capacity to walk up an escarpment in the frosty winter woods, to see their breath in the chilly air, or to feel the deep reward of vital exertion. We both hoped to help others avoid ever letting this happen.

Ultimately, however, this isn't within our control. It's up to every individual to make physical activity like this a way of life and a source of joy and pleasure. It's up to each and every one of us to bask in the invigoration and gratification that come from such physical exertion. Being physically active is part of who we are and how we are meant to be as human beings. And whether or not we appreciate that now, we would undoubtedly mourn the loss of these physical capabilities.

One of the best ways to learn to love the vitality that comes from physical activity has to do with being mindful—tuning in to your body's responses and soaking up the sensory stimuli from the environment you're moving in. If you can focus on how much stronger you feel from week to week or from month to month after sticking with an exercise program for a while, that's gratifying. If you pay attention to how vibrant and refreshed you feel after a brisk walk in fresh air or a good yoga class, that's a reward in itself, too. And if you can take note of the sounds of birds chirping in the trees or feel and enjoy the warmth of the sun on your face as you walk, jog, or snowshoe along a trail, the movement experience will be that much more enjoyable.

Continuing to feel grateful toward your body for allowing you to perform these physical feats becomes positive reinforcement to keep up the good work, too. Research from Germany found that when participants had positive experiences related to their exercise goals, they gained confidence that fostered more physical activity in the future. Whatever exercise-related measures we're inclined to pay attention to, I think we should all count our blessings if our limbs are working well and they're ready for action. Certainly those who don't have such blessings would see it that way.

Exercise in the most general sense—in the sense of movement—should not be a chore or a burden. It's a privilege, a source of joy, and a way to express our natural vitality. Nurture it, and it will nurture you. Squander it, and you will squander a critical opportunity to disease-proof yourself. Just as we can all love food that loves us back, the same is true of physical activity. With the right skillpower, we can each get health in the pursuit of pleasure and pleasure in the pursuit of health. If you accept that movement is something your body needs almost as much as it needs air, food, and water, then it comes down to choosing not *whether* to move your body, but how and when to do so.

THE DISEASE-PROOF TO-DO LIST:

- Embrace the benefits (to body and mind) of engaging in regular exercise by paying attention to improvements in how you feel and function.
- Pinpoint and cultivate your own motivation for becoming more active by challenging your reasons for not exercising.
- Identify physical activities that are in sync with your personality, preferences, and style.

- Learn how to frame a complete exercise program effectively, according to the FITT formula.
- Make time for workouts in your current schedule by treating them as important appointments or making them serve a dual purpose (as social events).
- Periodically shake up your routine to keep your workouts fresh, invigorating, and rewarding. This will ensure that you continue to challenge yourself physically and avoid the boredom or burnout that can derail your good exercise habits.
- Develop an appreciation for the vitality that comes from being physically active by enjoying the invigoration and sense of accomplishment that come from your physical feats.

• Eleven •

Nooks and Crannies: Finding Ways to Fit in Fitness

The Challenge: Physical activity takes time, and our modern schedules conspire against making movement routine.

The Right Response: Make regular physical activity a priority you are committed to fitting into your schedule, and seize any opportunity to slip more movement into your day.

The Relevant Skills: Using your muscles while you work; "doing the locomotion" whenever and wherever possible; making TV watching more active; taking up active hobbies that involve movement; and getting moving with your family and friends.

Words can be a bit like boots: Wear them around enough, and they tend to get dirty. There was a time when the word *exercise* evoked notions of fitness and vitality, good rewards for good effort. But little by little, the focus shifted to suffering and sweating. Health experts tried to create some positive spin by pointing out, "No pain, no gain!"—but too many people said, "Well, let's forget both, then!" Then we tried to change the response by noting that you can actually get physical fitness gains without pain. I'm not sure this approach worked, either. Exercise still sounds like something a lot of people want to avoid. But how about *play* or *sport* or *dance* or simply *healthy motion*? In recent decades, we've learned that all physical activity is good activity. It can, indeed, be sport or play; walking your dog or working in your garden counts. Playing tag or touch football with your children counts. Dancing counts, too!

It's easier than you may think to sneak more movement into your life. The basic idea is to fit exercise into your daily routine in increments that suit the available time, space, and occasion. For example, you can train yourself to take the stairs instead of making a beeline for the elevator or escalator in office and apartment buildings, shopping malls, or airports. You can walk on some of your errands instead of always driving. You can make everyday household chores more active just by doing them a little differently from usual—by raking instead of using a leaf blower, for example; washing your own car instead of going to a car wash; washing and drying dishes by hand rather than using the dishwasher. (Just because you have laborsaving technology doesn't mean you have to use it!) All this can make a difference in the big picture, because the benefits of moving more really do have a cumulative effect, and they start with the first step.

Throughout most of human history, vigorous daily activity was unavoidable, so there was probably a survival advantage for those who conserved energy when they could. As a result, we may well be *programmed* to cherish couch time. That was fine when exertion was obligatory and couches were nonexistent—but now the opposite is true. So if you want to be healthy, you have to outthink that obsolete Stone Age programming and get out there and move.

In the previous chapter, we laid out the building blocks for adopting a healthy exercise program that will help you disease-proof yourself. But life doesn't always obey your well-thought-out plans, and despite your good intentions, sometimes it just isn't possible to make time for a full exercise session. The good news is you don't need to make the perfect the enemy of the good. You can take steps to incorporate more movement into your day and still reap health benefits. And it doesn't have to be an either-or proposition: You can do both a full-fledged workout *and* include brief bursts of physical activity throughout your day for added benefits; or do one or the other on alternate days. This way, you'll boost your overall level of exercise and fitness *and* reduce the amount of time you spend sitting still. This is really the ideal scenario, because more movement is better.

When it comes right down to it, there really aren't any valid excuses for not moving more frequently throughout the day. On even the busiest of days, you brush your teeth and hair. You take a bath or shower. You put on deodorant. Some forms of self-care are simply automatic and nonnegotiable, no matter what. Physical activity deserves to be on that short list (for the reasons outlined in the previous chapter). If you think you don't have time to exercise, you almost certainly don't have time not to if you want to be the best, most upbeat, most intelligent, and efficient version of yourself! In the end, it comes down to this: You can invest time now in being healthy, or you can invest even more time later in being sick and having to take time off from work to lie in bed or go to doctors' appointments! (You also may not be able to keep up with your kids or grandkids or have an active retirement.) When you think of it this way, it's a pretty easy choice.

Chances are you'll come to enjoy physical activity as you make it a habit and adopt the right mind-set. In a series of four studies published in 2011, researchers at the University of British Columbia examined whether and why people tend to underestimate how much they enjoy physical activity. They found that across a broad range of exercise modalities—from yoga and Pilates to aerobic exercise and weight training—people significantly underestimated how much they would enjoy the activity, a phenomenon known as *forecasting myopia*. In a nutshell, people place a disproportionate emphasis on the beginning of an exercise session—when it tends to feel uncomfortable, maybe even unpleasant—rather than focusing on the middle or the end. In other words, they don't see the possibility of feeling vibrant, fully engaged, and strong during or after the workout. In the third and fourth studies, the researchers encouraged the participants to *expect* to enjoy their movement sessions—and it worked! Better still, it increased the participants' intention to exercise.

Small Changes, Big Payoffs

Sadly, in our culture it is now considered fairly normal to get diabetes or heart disease as we age. It is routine to develop high blood pressure, insulin resistance, and high cholesterol and to end up taking a slew of medications. None of these scenarios needs to happen. Many of my patients who are at retirement age have invested over the years to ensure some degree of financial security. Most of them achieve it and have the financial means to travel and live as they'd like to. But along the way, too many of them failed to treat health and fitness as equally as important as wealth. The result was they did not have the physical security or fortitude to fully enjoy their retirement opportunities. The fact is that even modest investments in fitness and conditioning pay incredible dividends, by reducing the risk of developing major chronic diseases.

Fortunately, we have come to recognize that just about any way of fitting in exercise is good. It needn't be in one long bout, and we needn't all make the Olympic team. Brief bursts of exercise that add up to a reasonable dose (thirty minutes) over the course of the day will do just fine, as will moderate-intensity exercise. As Gretchen Reynolds notes in her book *The First 20 Minutes*, numerous studies suggest that nearly all the reductions in mortality stem from the first twenty minutes of exercise; after that, it's basically icing on the proverbial cake, as far as longevity goes, though you'll continue to derive additional health benefits.

In 2006, colleagues and I developed ABC for Fitness, a free physical activity program for kids to use in school or at home, and a program, called Activity Bursts Everywhere (ABE for Fitness) for adults to use at work. ABC for Fitness includes warm-up, aerobic, and cool-down calisthenic and dance moves that kids can do in a classroom right next to their desks. By contrast, ABE for Fitness offers a library of online videos for stretching, calisthenic, and isometric exercises adults can do next to their desks or, in some cases, even while seated at them! Both allow for intermittent, brief bursts of high-quality physical activity throughout the day. We have proven results, too: Our study of ABC for Fitness in three schools in Missouri found that it improved fitness measures, health, and behavior—without interfering with reading, writing, and arithmetic.

There are also options for converting work at a desk from a sitting to a walking activity for those who are so inclined. Research from the Mayo Clinic found that when people walk in place while they work, they burn nearly 120 calories more per hour than when they do the same tasks seated. Doing this for two hours a day, without changing your eating habits, could add up to significant weight loss over the course of a year, as well as substantial health benefits.

You don't necessarily have to join a gym or become a hardcore fitness enthusiast to reap the benefits of regular physical activity. Instead, simply choose to move regularly throughout the day. How? By lifting dumbbells, using resistance bands, or riding an exercise bike while you watch TV instead of sitting still. Take a walk on a lunchtime errand instead of driving. Meet a friend for a walk or a bike ride instead of for coffee. Dance with your kids when you come home from work. The notion that formal *exercise* is the only way to derive benefits from physical activity is yesterday's news. Simple levels of physical activity are enormously beneficial. So during the day, seize any opportunity to use muscle power instead of relying on technology—and you'll be doing your health a world of good.

The Skill: Using Your Muscles While You Work

Who says you need to sit at your desk in order to get work done? If you set up your work environment accordingly, you can do it just as well from a standing position. When you stand, you recruit different muscles to stay upright, which helps burn more calories. In fact, research from Miami University in Ohio found that when people performed reading and speech tasks while standing at an "active workstation," their metabolic rate increased significantly (by a factor of three!) from when they did the same tasks seated—and there was no deterioration in their speech quality. If you have the option to work at a vertical workstation that allows you to walk on a treadmill while working on a computer, that's even better.

You can also swap your desk chair for a stability ball. Researchers at the State University of New York at Buffalo ran a study in which people performed clerical work in various postures, and compared the amount of energy they expended during each. When the participants performed the work while sitting on a stability ball or standing, they burned 4 additional calories per hour than they did while sitting on a desk chair. The calorie-burning effects were comparable between the stability ball and standing postures, but the participants liked sitting on the ball more (as much as a desk chair). It's not a big jump in calories burned, but you'll also be using more of the muscles in your core (your abdomen, hips, and back) to support yourself on the stability ball, which is a good thing! To sit on a fitness ball correctly, make a conscious effort to sit up straight, pull your belly button in toward your spine, and squeeze your shoulder blades together behind you; also, keep your head in line with your neck and spine. (No slouching allowed!)

From the *Things-You-Never-Knew-You-Never-Knew* Files

There's no shame in fidgeting. In fact, fidgeting (which falls under the umbrella of non-exercise activity thermogenesis, or NEAT, in research parlance) burns more calories than being still does, according to research from the Mayo Clinic. So go ahead and jiggle your feet while you're sitting, and shift your weight from one foot to the other while you're standing in line.

The Skill: "Doing the Locomotion" Whenever and Wherever Possible

It's as simple as this: Whenever you have the chance, put your feet to good use by walking. If you have children, walk them to the bus stop or part of the way to school in the mornings. If you take a lunch break, use your feet to take you wherever you need to go to buy your lunch; if you're brown-bagging it, take a brisk walk to clear your mind and boost your circulation before or after you eat. These are simple, easy steps—and they matter!

If you have a dog, make it a point to walk it at least a couple of times per day. In a recent study, researchers at the George Washington University School of Public Health and Health Services, in Washington, D.C., assessed the differences in levels of physical activity and risk factors between dog owners who walk their dogs, those who don't, and people who don't own dogs: The dog walkers had a lower BMI as well as a lower prevalence of diabetes, hypertension, high cholesterol, and depression. If you don't have a dog, and it's compatible with your lifestyle, consider getting one. In a study comparing the physical activity levels between 351 dog owners and those without dogs, researchers from the University of Victoria, in Canada, found that those with canine companions walked an average of 132 minutes more per week than non-dog owners did. If owning a dog isn't an option for you, offer to walk a friend's or neighbor's dog, or make it a point to regularly walk with your spouse, children, or a friend, or even by yourself, through your neighborhood or to a park.

Whenever you go to appointments, shopping malls, or even your own office building, park farther away from the door instead of looking for the closest spot. When you get inside, use the stairs instead of the elevator or escalator. Stair-climbing is a high-intensity, efficient form of physical activity that builds aerobic fitness and muscle and bone strength in your legs, reduces levels of harmful cholesterol, and burns extra calories. When researchers at the University Hospital of Geneva, in Switzerland, ran a promotional campaign for stair use by employees of the hospital, the number of one-story climbs and descents on the stairs rose from 4.5 per day to 20.6 per day—a fourfold increase! After twelve weeks, the participants were fitter (as measured by maximal aerobic capacity) and had experienced significant declines in waist circumference, body fat, diastolic blood pressure, and low-density lipoprotein, or LDL (the "bad," artery-clogging) cholesterol. An easy way to make taking the stairs a habit is to follow the two up, three down guideline: Whenever you need to go two floors up or three floors down in a building, choose the stairs instead of the elevator. It takes only a matter of minutes, and that's really the point—you can give your health a boost with every bout of movement, even if it's brief.

If you want to see how it adds up throughout the day—or if you want a specific goal to work toward—consider getting a pedometer. A recent study from Brazil found that physically inactive smokers who wore a pedometer every day for a month increased their daily steps by an average of 2,640 steps—and they were able to walk farther in a six-minute walking test than at the beginning of the study, which is proof positive that they achieved fitness gains. Becoming more physically active also helped them cut back on their daily cigarettes. Similarly, researchers from Saint Louis University, in Missouri, found that when adults age sixty-five and older wore a pedometer every day for four weeks, they increased their daily step count by 23 percent.

To increase your step count, and your overall physical activity, it's also wise to use *active transportation* as often as possible. This means walking or bicycling for transportation, a practice that pays off generously in the health department. In a study published in 2012 in the *American Journal of Preventive Medicine*, researchers examined the relationship between active transportation and risk factors for cardiovascular disease in more than 9,900 adults in the United States and found that the vast majority (76 percent!) didn't use active transportation. Among those who did, BMI and mean waist circumference were lower compared with those who didn't use active transportation; even more impressively, those with high levels of active transportation were 31 percent less likely to have hypertension or diabetes.

Granted, it's not possible for everyone to walk or bike to work; many of us work in cities or towns that are many miles away from our homes. But we can all use our feet to get us places at other times. The point is it pays (in health dividends) to think about using your feet instead of your car whenever possible. Why drive someplace when it's possible to walk or bike there instead? A bit more muscle power and a bit less fossil fuel also happen to be good for the planet.

The Skill: Making TV Watching More Active

There's no law of the universe that says you must be planted on your bottom on the couch in order to watch TV. You can enjoy your favorite shows while riding a stationary bike, walking on a treadmill, or using an elliptical machine. Even just using commercial breaks as an opportunity to move your body—perhaps by jumping rope or doing jumping jacks—can make a difference. A recent study at the University of Tennessee, Knoxville, found that stepping in place during commercials nearly doubles a person's calorie expenditure while watching TV for an hour. Another recent study published in the *International Journal of Behavioral Nutrition and Physical Activity* found that when participants briskly stepped in place or walked around the room during commercials, while watching at least ninety minutes of TV at least five days per week, they experienced significant reductions in body fat as well as waist and hip circumference after six months. It's a minimal commitment that doesn't detract from enjoyment of your regularly scheduled program. You can also sneak in a strength-training workout while you watch TV, using dumbbells, resistance bands, or your own body weight. Drop to the ground and do a set of push-ups, triceps dips, crunches, bicycle crunches, and the plank. Or stay on your feet and do sets of different squats (basic squats, plié squats, wide squats, wall squats, and so on), followed by forward and reverse lunges.

As you can see, you don't need your own home gym, but it's a good idea to have some basic exercise gear on hand so you can do strength-training moves at home, at the park, or even when you travel. This includes a jump rope, resistance bands (which come in varying degrees of tension), hand-held weights (from 2.5 to 15.0 pounds), and a stability ball. Just make sure to buy the right-size ball for your height: 55 centimeters if you're 5 feet 3 inches or shorter; 65 centimeters if you're 5 feet 4 to 5 feet 10; and 75 centimeters if you're 5 feet 11 or taller. You can use it as a weight bench (to do chest presses, for example), or to make abdominal exercises more challenging.

The Skill: Taking Up Active Hobbies That Involve Movement

There's a fertile middle ground for movement between exercise and relatively still hobbies such as reading, painting, or cooking. Whether you take up gardening, woodworking, rock climbing, martial arts, tango dancing, or bird-watching (assuming you'll be hiking into the woods), you'll be using your body as a critical tool in creating a sense of enjoyment. This is a vital aspect of what Mihaly Csikszentmihalyi, PhD, calls "flow" (in his book by the same name)—a state of optimal experience in which someone is concentrating so intently on an activity that she becomes completely immersed or absorbed in it.

Elite athletes often refer to this phenomenon as "being in the zone." Runners call it the "runners' high," but it's something everyone can attain with enough of a challenge at the right intensity. In that state, time becomes irrelevant; the person's worries and self-consciousness vanish into the ether. Besides gaining a tremendous sense of satisfaction and enjoyment from doing such activities, the time during which you're engaged in them is likely to pass quickly, which may inspire you to do them for longer or to seek out more opportunities to do them. It's all to the good, really, because this positively reinforces keeping up the rewarding work.

As we discussed in the last chapter, discovering active hobbies and physical activities that create that optimal experience for you may involve some trial and error. But it helps if you find activities that require learning skills, setting up goals, getting feedback about how you're doing, and allowing for a sense of control. These are the critical elements that will allow you to become fully immersed and engaged in what you're doing. Research from the Nanyang Technological University, in Japan, suggests that achieving an ongoing state of flow depends most highly on engaging in physical activities that strike a balance between being challenging and being manageable with one's skills. Tilt the balance too far in one direction or the other—meaning the activity is either too difficult or not challenging enough—and it's less likely to produce that optimal experience. Try to find activities that you truly enjoy, that help you build skills, and that are just right in the challenge department. After that, the stage has been set, and it's up to you to get your head in the game.

An added benefit of hobby-related activities is that it's a great opportunity to meet people with a similar interest, and make friends. Speaking of which . . .

The Skill: Getting Moving with Your Family and Friends

My wife, Catherine, is a social exerciser. Don't get me wrong: She's committed to physical activity, but given the choice, she finds it more fun to do it with other people, and having the distraction of other people's company helps the time pass faster for her. Whenever we go for a long walk or hike and we encounter a hill, it's my job to provide entertaining banter all the way up the incline.

The best way to make exercise a social experience will vary with your personal circumstances. It can mean taking a class, such as yoga, Zumba, kickboxing, or Spinning; going on hikes or bike rides with family members or friends; or playing tag or Frisbee or having dance contests with your kids. It can also mean joining a recreational sports team (soccer, volleyball, or softball, for example) or entering a round robin for tennis or squash.

The social component adds more than just the pleasure of camaraderie and a pleasant distraction from the physical exertion; it also adds an element of accountability. Your exercise buddies will come to count on you to show up, just as you count on them to do the same. This accountability to others is a form of *social contracting* (in the parlance of the behavior change circles), and studies have found that it really does boost adherence to exercise. In one study, researchers at Indiana University found that adults who joined an exercise program with a spouse were 35 percent more likely to attend regularly and nearly seven times less likely to drop out after a year than married people who took the solo route.

How you make physical activity social is entirely up to you. The options are limitless. And you don't have to make it social all the time; doing so occasionally, with solo exercise sessions in between, may provide an appealing balance.

Your Usual Day—with More Movement

Wake-up: Do some easy stretches in bed, followed by abdominal crunches or the plank.

Fit in a morning aerobic workout if possible.

Have a healthy breakfast.

Go to work; take the stairs when you get there.

Lunchtime: Have a healthy lunch then take a brief walk.

Midafternoon: Do stretches at your desk or strengthening moves such as squats or triceps dips (using a stable chair without wheels).

After work: Fit in an aerobic workout if you didn't in the A.M., meet a friend for an exercise class, or take a walk or bike ride.

Have a healthy dinner.

Evening: Move during commercials and do strengthening exercises while watching TV.

In the grand scheme of life, getting to 30 minutes of physical activity each day is not a big hill to climb. It's a worthy investment in your health and well-being, for today and tomorrow. Think of it this way: There are 1,440 minutes in every day; of that total, 20 minutes represents less than 1.4 percent. If a day were a dollar, for a penny and half of it you could pay to keep diabetes away. (Of course, there's not an absolute guarantee, but nothing else even comes close to this sort of return on investment.) So stop coming up with excuses and start moving more.

Edward is a former patient of mine who has struggled with his weight for much of his adult life. He continues to frequently check in with me, asking for my opinion on the latest diet book du jour. In recent years my advice to him has been consistent: Stop reading and get off the couch! To his credit, he has (finally) stopped seeking the magic cure-all in any given diet and has taken up hiking with a passion, which has helped him shed 18 pounds and improve his health. I'm impressed, and proud of him, because he learned a lesson that's important for us all: In so many ways, getting physical really is the best thing we can do for ourselves.

It's time, then, to turn our habits on their head. Instead of exercising for thirty to sixty minutes per day and sitting the rest of the time, we should reverse this pattern. In addition to exercising, stand up every thirty to sixty minutes—or at least every couple of hours—and walk around, move around, or do something else to break up those long sedentary stretches! Instead of aiming to get the bare minimum of movement in a day, seek opportunities for more. It's time to recapture the natural proclivity for movement that's within all human beings. We really do need to move our bodies—regularly!—if we don't want to risk losing their vitality and health.

The Nooks and Crannies Workout

Here's a simple strength-training workout that includes different moves to strengthen the muscles in your upper body, your core, and your lower body. You can do them at home, while watching TV or waiting for dinner to cook in the oven, or even during your lunch break. Some of the moves require just your own body weight; others use resistance bands or dumbbells. Choose an exercise from each category and move through each category before returning to the first one and repeating the cycle. (This way, you'll end up doing two sets of each exercise.) To challenge as many different muscles as possible, include at least two different exercises from each category (at least two sets of six different exercises). Ready, set, get to it!

Upper Body

Triceps dips: Stand in front of a sturdy chair or bench, bend your legs as if you were about to sit down, and place your palms with fingers facing forward on the seat's front edge, shoulder width apart. Your feet should be flat on the ground in front of you, with your arms supporting most of your body weight. Bend your arms and slowly lower your body until your elbows are bent at a ninety-degree angle and your hips drop toward the floor in front of the seat. Pause, then return to the starting position. Do twelve to fifteen reps.

Push-ups: Lie facedown with your legs straight, your feet slightly apart, and the balls of your feet on the floor. Place your palms on the floor slightly more than shoulder-width apart and in line with your chest muscles. Straighten your arms so you push your body off the floor, keeping your belly muscles engaged, your neck and head in line with your spine, your chest lifted, and your body as straight as a board. Bend your arms and lower your body toward the floor as far as you can, then push yourself back up to the start position. Do twelve to fifteen reps. (If you have trouble doing full push-ups, do modified push-ups: Start in the position just described, but with knees on the floor and feet lifted.)

Bicep curls (with resistance band or dumbbells): If you're using a resistance band, stand on the midsection of the band, with your feet hip-width apart and hold the handles of the resistance band with your palms facing up. Start with your arms straight by your sides, then bend your elbows and bring your palms up toward your shoulders, then lower your arms. Do a set of twelve to fifteen reps. If you're using dumbbells, hold one in each hand, with palms facing up, and do the same move.

Upright rows (with resistance band or dumbbells): If you're using a resistance band, stand on the midsection of the band with your feet hip-width apart and hold the handles of the resistance band with your palms facing your thighs. Keeping your head and chest lifted, engage your abdominal muscles, and bend your elbows as you pull the band's handles straight up to collarbone level so your elbows point out to the sides; return to start. Do twelve to fifteen reps. If you're using dumbbells, use the same motion while holding a dumbbell in each hand with your thumbs facing your body.

Shoulder presses (with dumbbells): Stand with your feet shoulder-width apart, one foot slightly in front of the other to protect your lower back. Hold a dumbbell in each hand just above shoulder level, with your palms facing forward and your elbows pointing toward the ground. Press your arms up overhead until your elbows are fully extended; return to the start position. Do twelve to fifteen reps.

Core

Abdominal crunches: Lie on your back with bent knees. Place your feet flat on the floor hip-width apart. Place your hands behind your head with your elbows open wide and parallel to the floor. Lift your shoulder blades off the floor, keeping your chin off your chest and pressing your lower back against the floor as you rise. Pause at the top and then slowly lower your shoulders to the floor. Do twelve to fifteen reps.

Plank: Lie facedown on the floor and raise yourself onto your forearms and toes so your elbows are right under your chest. Keep your hips raised, your back flat, and your neck in line with your spine; your body should resemble a "plank" that's parallel to the floor. Pull your belly button toward your spine to engage the abdominal muscles. Hold this position for thirty seconds, then relax. Do three reps, gradually working up to holding the move for sixty seconds.

Side plank: This exercise targets the oblique muscles along the sides of your abdomen. Lie on your left side with your shoulders, hips, knees, and feet aligned and your feet stacked on top of each other. Raise yourself onto your left forearm with your left shoulder directly above your left elbow and balance on your forearm and the side of your left (lower) foot; your right arm can rest along the right side of your body. Hold this position for ten seconds, then release. Do ten reps. Then roll onto your right side and repeat.

Shoulder bridge: To strengthen the muscles in your pelvis, thighs, abdomen, and butt, lie on your back with your knees bent and your feet flat on the floor. Extend your arms out to the sides near shoulder level for balance. Slowly lift your hips high enough off the floor so that only your shoulder blades and shoulders remain on the floor; pause, then slowly return your hips to the floor. Do twelve to fifteen reps.

Bicycle crunches: Lie on your back. Extend your legs and lift them a few inches off the floor with your hands behind your head, elbows open wide. In a fluid motion: bend your right knee and bring it toward your upper body (keeping the left leg straight) as you twist your torso so that your left elbow nearly touches your right knee; then twist and repeat the motion with opposing limbs. Do twelve to fifteen reps.

Lower Body

Side-lying upper-leg raises: Lie on your right side with your legs stacked and your body in a straight line from your head to your toes. Bend your right arm and rest your head in your right hand; place your left hand on the floor in front of you for support. Tighten your abdominal muscles and slowly lift your left leg as high as you can comfortably, with your foot flexed. Pause for a second, then lower your leg. Do twelve to fifteen reps, then turn onto your left side and repeat with the right leg.

Side-lying lower-leg raises: Lie on your right side with your legs stacked and your body in a straight line from your head to your toes. Bend your right arm and rest your head in your right hand; place your left hand on the floor in front of you for support. Bend your left leg and bring your left foot onto the floor in front of your right thigh. Tighten your abdominal muscles and slowly lift your right leg off the floor, keeping your foot flexed and your body steady. Pause for a second at the top, then lower your right leg. Do twelve to fifteen reps, then turn onto your left side and repeat with the left leg.

The Duck Walk (with resistance band): Place both feet on a resistance band, shoulder-width apart, so the band is under the balls of your feet. Cross the band in front of you and grab a handle with each hand, holding it at hip level (there should be tension in the band). With knees slightly bent, step to the right with your right foot, keeping the band taut, then bring your left foot toward your right so your feet are shoulder-width apart again. Take ten to fifteen steps to the right; then switch sides and walk ten to fifteen steps to the left.

The Penguin (with resistance band): Start in the same position as the Duck Walk but instead of stepping to the side, you'll be stepping forward and back. With your feet shoulder-width apart (and tension in the band) and your spine straight, step forward 8–12 inches with your right foot, then step forward with your left so your left foot is parallel to your right; next, step 8–12 inches back with your right foot, then do it with your left. Do ten to fifteen reps.

Squats (with or without dumbbells): Stand with your feet shoulder-width apart and your arms at your sides. As you bend your knees, place your weight on your heels and lower your butt as if you were going to sit in a chair, while raising your arms out in front of you for balance. As you do this, be sure to keep your back straight and your feet parallel. Your knees should not extend over your toes. Return to the start position; do twelve to fifteen reps. For an extra challenge, do squats while holding a dumbbell in each hand at your sides.

THE DISEASE-PROOF TO-DO LIST:

- Engage more muscles at work. Instead of sitting like a statue, move your body or involve more muscle groups in your day job.
- Do the locomotion whenever you get the chance. Every step adds up to more physical activity over the course of a day. Rely on your feet (rather than machines) more often for transportation.
- Turn TV time into more active time and you'll easily combine pleasure with movement.
- Cultivate some hobbies that involve movement, not just sitting.
- Incorporate physical activity into leisure time with your family and friends by making formal exercise social or by finding other ways to get moving together.

• Twelve •

The Whole(istic) Truth

The prize of enhanced health and greater longevity requires a working understanding of the science of disease prevention, a reasonable dose of good sense, and the ability to see the big picture. By now you're well aware of the science that illustrates how better use of our feet and forks can slash our risk of developing chronic diseases and how health-promoting habits can even influence the expression of our genes in positive ways. And we know that you've got good sense, because you've already taken a big step toward disease-proofing yourself by reading this book!

Good sense often suggests what is likely to be true, blazing trails that scientific inquiry follows in order to verify (or refute) what solid hypotheses have suggested. Good sense also tells us that if something sounds too good to be true, it almost certainly is. The only real problem with good common sense is that it isn't used commonly enough, particularly when it comes to achieving weight loss and better health.

The third element, the big picture, is something we often miss entirely. We fail to see the forest for the trees. It happens when we go looking for the quick fix that will make us thin, fit, or healthy, and when we mistake some dietary supplement for a substitute for eating well or exercising regularly.

One of my patients, Denise, forty-five, initially came to see me because she wanted help losing weight, but we needed to consider the big picture first. At 5 feet 3 and 192 pounds, with a BMI of 34, she had both high blood pressure and type 2 diabetes. Her excess body fat was a contributing factor, if not the outright cause, of both conditions. She was taking medications for her diabetes and hypertension, and she complained of their side effects. The side effects weren't bad enough for her to stop taking the drugs, but they made her feel a bit rundown all the time. Denise also took anti-inflammatory medications for arthritis in her knees and hips. The arthritis was largely due to her excess weight, which had stressed her joints for many years. She knew she should exercise, but whenever she tried, her joints would ache, so she had abandoned exercise altogether, which naturally had led to more weight gain. And, of course, the heavier she got, the more stress she put on her joints, worsening the arthritis.

Complicating matters, Denise slept poorly and typically woke up many times each night. Her husband, with whom she had a strained relationship, was sleeping in a separate bedroom, partly because they weren't getting along and partly because both of them snored. Because Denise never slept well, she was always tired, frequently irritable, and lacked both the motivation and the restraint to eat better or exercise. She was also lonely, sad, and felt pretty discouraged overall.

In other words, Denise was stuck in a vicious cycle where she was eating too much of the wrong foods, partly because she was often hungry but partly because eating gave her the pleasure she was missing in other areas of her life. Overeating made her weight go up and her joints hurt more; the quality of her sleep kept going down, while the amount of medication she needed to control her joint pain, blood pressure, and blood sugar continued to go up. Theoretically, Denise wanted me to give her dietary counseling so she could lose weight, but there was a whole lot more to her story than that. We needed to consider the big picture.

In medicine, holistic care has been defined as "a system of comprehensive or total patient care that considers the physical, emotional, social, economic, and spiritual needs of the person; his or her response to illness; and the effect of the illness on the ability to meet self-care needs." In theory, I am comfortable with this definition. In practice, not so much. Here's why: This definition begs the questions: How exactly do you do that in a doctor-patient encounter? What's a clinician actually supposed to do in an examining room to address all a patient's health needs in one fell swoop? Holistic care is hardest to do when there's a lot that needs fixing, as in Denise's case.

When a patient's condition is going from bad to worse, especially a seriously ill patient who's in the hospital, doctors tend to talk about that person "circling the drain." (Medical jargon can be a bit uncouth; on behalf of my profession, I apologize for that.) What this means in simple terms is that a complex array of medical, emotional, and social problems really can resemble a cascade in which each malady worsens another, and the net effect is a downward spiral into despondent disability or imminent death. "Circling the drain" is a crude but apt metaphor. Denise was experiencing this phenomenon, even though she wasn't (yet) terminally ill.

Think of it this way: If we can approach the drain one health problem at a time, it follows that we can climb back out from it and ascend a spiral staircase toward vitality in just the same way. In other words, any given health *problem* can make others worse, but any given health *solution* can help make that one problem and others better. In my view, that is what holistic care needs to be. This is true when you are receiving care from your doctor and it's also true when you are providing the care yourself. When a doctor provides care, each solution may be some kind of therapy. When you are troubleshooting on your own, each solution is apt to be based on a skill.

In Denise's case, we had to figure out together which was the first key health factor that needed to be addressed. For her, the priority was to (finally!) get a good night's sleep. So I ordered a formal sleep study, which revealed that she had sleep apnea, a chronic disorder that causes repeated pauses in breathing while the person sleeps. When we got her sleep apnea under good control—there are various ways to do this—she slept through the night for the first time in years and began feeling more energetic, more encouraged, and more motivated about her well-being. She was also less hungry, her mood was more stable, and her joints hurt a bit less.

The deal I made with Denise was this: Each time we made some progress with one of her issues, she would "invest" it back into her overall health. What this meant was that the increased energy and decreased joint pain she gained presented an opportunity to start some gentle exercise. For Denise, that meant walking slowly. (For other patients with joint pain, water aerobics can be a good option.) We then addressed the joint pain directly—with massage therapy for osteoarthritis of her knees—and it helped. She was able to cut back on her pain medication. Since having less joint pain meant she could walk more, she did—and gradually she started to lose weight. Little by little, this reduced the stress on her joints.

At my suggestion, Denise and her husband started couples' therapy, where they addressed issues they had long left smoldering. Since then, their relationship has improved substantially and is now increasingly based on mutual support, respect, and affection. It is becoming a source of strength for them both, instead of a source of stress. And Denise's husband has joined her in eating more healthfully, becoming more active, and gaining better health, using the same skill set that's been laid out in this book. Over a two-year period, Denise has lost 60 pounds and reversed her type 2 diabetes, her hypertension, and her sleep apnea. She gets an occasional massage for much milder joint pain and very occasionally takes ibuprofen. She sleeps well most nights and has energy to invest in living better.

By any measure, she has ascended from the drain of related diseases, and climbed her way toward better health. Our initial appointment was supposed to be about weight, but there was much more to Denise's situation. I'm delighted to say, it's a story with a happy ending—one that's far more accessible than most people realize.

Health is, inescapably, holistic, a complete package. (After all, being healthy on your left side doesn't matter if there's a tumor on your right.) It's the whole package that matters most, yet each of the contributing elements can influence every other. You need to know how to shop for healthy ingredients before you can begin cooking healthy meals, and you need to know how to expand or reform your taste buds' repertoire if you want to train your palate to prefer good nutrition. You need to identify physical activities that you enjoy, but you also need to find ways to work them into your busy life.

This dynamic, which I call *skill synergy*, is a common phenomenon within other disciplines. When learning a foreign language, the more words and phrases you master, the easier it becomes to master the rest. As a carpenter, each tool you learn to use makes learning to use the next one easier, because many of the skills that are required cross over from one tool to another. The same is true for healthy living.

By reading this book, you are well on your way to mastering all the different skills and creating skill synergy. To take it to the next level, you'll want to personalize the approach you take in building your own Skill Spiral, by starting with the skills that are most essential or applicable to you and tending to the supporting elements that will make it easier or more comfortable for you to adjust your eating and movement habits. Before you can tailor your approach to eating more healthfully and exercising more regularly, you'll want to take stock of other aspects of your lifestyle that can help or hinder your efforts. Among the most important influences are: the quality and quantity of your sleep, how much stress you experience and how well (or poorly) you manage it, whether you're in chronic pain, and the state of your relationships.

The Upside of Downtime: Sound Sleep

The quality and quantity of your sleep has profound effects on your body and mind, psychologically, immunologically, and neurologically. One of the effects of chronic sleep deprivation is that it lowers the pain threshold; in other words, everything that hurts aches more when you're sleep deprived. Sleep also influences every organ system in the body; it's while you're snoozing that the body does most of its regenerative work. Moreover, sleep directly affects our brain waves. So when sleep is disrupted, fragmented, or insufficient, our brain wave patterns can get out of sync with our lifestyles. We may experience brain waves that are conducive to sleep when we're trying to work and be productive, and brain waves that are appropriate for thinking and other mentally challenging activities when we're trying to fall asleep. This can take a serious toll on the quality of our lives. While extreme sleep deprivation can be lethal, even milder disruptions in healthy brain wave patterns can cause irritability, impatience, difficulty concentrating, frustration, anger, and depression.

Inadequate slumber over extended periods of time also may interfere with immune function, including the proper production of white blood cells and hormonal regulation, which is why insufficient sleep is linked with chronically elevated levels of the stress hormone cortisol. This also leads to impaired immunity and elevated levels of hormones such as insulin, increasing the risk of gaining body fat (most often in the midsection) and of developing systemic inflammation and type 2 diabetes. It also leads to changes in the hormones leptin and ghrelin, which regulate hunger and satiety.

From the *Things-You-Never-Knew-You-Never-Knew* Files

Research has found a link between sleep, the body's circadian rhythms (the twenty-four-hour fluctuations in hormone levels), energy regulation (including hunger), and obesity all the way down to the level of our genes. Sleep deprivation can change gene expression for the bad; sleeping better can change it for the good!

On top of these direct effects, changing behavior is challenging and requires both willpower and skillpower, both of which depend on having sufficient amounts of energy. As you undoubtedly know from personal experience, when you're exhausted or you feel depleted, you probably don't feel motivated to do much of anything. Well, chronic sleep deprivation and/or chronic sleep disturbances can make those feelings a permanent state of affairs, eroding your motivation and dissolving your resolve to eat more healthfully or be more active. Plus, if you're sleep deprived, you're apt to be irritable and hungry, and you're more likely to turn to food for comfort. All of this can set into motion a toxic cycle, because making poor food choices, gaining weight, and being sedentary can interfere with good-quality sleep!

Here are some tips to help you get onto more solid ground:

- **Maintain a consistent sleep schedule.** This means stick with the same bedtime and awakening time (or within an hour of the same) every day of the week, even on the weekends.
- **Avoid napping during the day.** It's okay to take a twenty- to thirty-minute nap occasionally if you're exhausted and you need to refresh yourself, but go beyond that and you're likely to interfere with your sleep that night.
- **Steer clear of stimulants too close to bedtime.** These include caffeine, nicotine (which you should be avoiding anyway), and alcohol. While consuming alcohol can make you sleepy at first, it can disrupt sleep in the second half of the night as your body metabolizes it. So don't have caffeine after 3:00 P.M. (before noon if you're very sensitive to its effects) and keep your alcohol intake in the moderate zone (one to two drinks).
- **Exercise regularly during the day.** Whether you work out in the morning or afternoon is up to you; just don't do vigorous exercise within four hours of bedtime or it may keep you up (yoga or Pilates shouldn't be a problem in the evening).
- **Establish a relaxing routine before turning in.** That can mean taking a warm bath, reading an enjoyable book, listening to music, or doing some gentle stretches. Try to avoid emotionally charged conversations or activities (such as watching the news) before bed. Don't bring stress and worries to bed with you.
- **Make sure your bedroom is conducive to sleep.** Don't do work

or watch TV in bed. Your bedroom should be quiet and dark. Your bed should be comfortable, and the room shouldn't be too hot or too cold.

- **Consult your doctor.** If your sleep troubles persist, there may be more going on than meets the eye. Your doctor can help you figure it out.

The Strain of Excess Stress

Many of the negative effects of insufficient sleep also occur with chronic stress. The resulting hormonal imbalances (involving cortisol and insulin, in particular) and chronic low-grade inflammation can set the stage for the development of heart disease, type 2 diabetes, some forms of cancer, and other chronic diseases. Chronic stress can also make you more susceptible to colds, flus, and other infections. And psychological stress disrupts physiological homeostasis in a number of ways (including the hormonal and inflammatory pathways) that may affect your energy level in an adverse way.

It can also affect your state of mind, impairing your working memory and your ability to control your impulses and increasing the risk of anxiety and depression. And unbridled stress can sap your energy and undermine your motivation and resolve to make or stick with healthy lifestyle changes. In fact, research from the University of California, San Francisco, found that people who reported higher levels of stress had a greater drive to eat, including disinhibited eating, binge eating, hunger, and more ineffective attempts to control their eating, all of which can promote weight gain.

To get the upper hand on stress, try the following strategies:

- **Develop better time-management skills.** Prioritize what needs to be done as soon as you can get to it, then address tasks and responsibilities that are next in line, while putting on the back burner those that can wait for a while.

- **Lighten your plate of responsibilities.** Learn to say no to nonessential requests, and delegate tasks that can be easily fulfilled by other people (such as family members or colleagues).
- **Give yourself breathing lessons.** Learn to breathe slowly and rhythmically—in through your nose (for a count of three) and out through your mouth (for a count of three). This can make stress less distressing. Whenever you feel stress getting the best of you, take a time-out and breathe deeply.
- **Exercise regularly.** Besides bathing your brain and body in feel-good neurotransmitters (such as serotonin), physical activity will help you feel more empowered to handle what's happening in your life.
- **Discover your optimal tension-taming technique.** It could be meditation, progressive muscle relaxation, visualization, or another technique. Through trial and error, find what works for you and use it regularly.
- **Give yourself a thought makeover.** The way you think about stress can make it better or worse. So stop negative thinking habits—such as looking at the worst-case scenario, engaging in all-or-nothing thinking, or taking things personally—in their tracks and try to find a more neutral way to think about what's happening. Challenge your negative thoughts by asking yourself how likely it is that your worst fear will actually happen, avoiding extreme words such as *always* and *never*, and asking yourself whether you have evidence that what you're saying to yourself is actually true.
- **Practice good self-care.** You should be doing this as a matter of habit, but it's especially important when you're under stress to eat a healthy diet, get plenty of sleep, exercise regularly, and limit your alcohol and caffeine consumption.

A personal comment about stress management: In my clinic, we deal with this all the time and routinely refer patients to interventions such as yoga, meditation, visualization, and breathing exercises—with good effect. This might work for you, too. What works to clear *my* head is vigorous activity, preferably outdoors—hiking, a walk with my dogs, some time riding my horse Troubadour. The point is simply: What works for you is what works for you! When it comes to stress relief, that ancient adage *know thyself* is really where progress starts. Pick the approach that feels right to you. Just don't neglect your stress!

The Drain of Chronic Pain

Whether it's constant, intermittent, or recurring, when you have chronic pain, it's hard to feel motivated to change your behavior or to have the energy to do so. It can be hard to sleep well or manage stress. Moreover, chronic pain can have a negative trickle-down effect on various aspects of your lifestyle, often leading to insomnia, stress overload, depression, relationship problems, lack of exercise, and poor dietary choices. Chronic pain, particularly joint pain, headaches, back and neck pain, is an incredibly common problem—more than 100 million adults in the United States suffer from it, according to the Institute of Medicine—and it's one of the most common reasons people visit their doctors.

For the sake of your health and well-being, it's essential to work closely with your doctor to get your pain under good control. Most people with chronic pain will benefit from a multidimensional approach, involving medications (such as opioids, analgesics, anti-inflammatory drugs, or antidepressants), topical agents (ranging from capsaicin cream to lidocaine or nonsteroidal anti-inflammatory patches), mind-body approaches (such as cognitive-behavioral therapy, biofeedback, relaxation training, and mindfulness meditation), and rehabilitative approaches (such as physical therapy, occupational therapy, and the application of heat or cold). For many types of pain, complementary techniques such as acupuncture, therapeutic massage, and yoga have been found to help, too.

The first step is to:

- **Be specific in describing the pain.** Tell your doctor where the pain is located, when it started, whether it's constant or it waxes and wanes, and what provokes or eases it. Provide details about what it feels like (whether it's a stabbing, throbbing, burning sensation or a dull ache, for example). It can also help to describe the pain's intensity on a scale from one to ten (with ten being the worst pain you can imagine).

- **Describe how the pain is impacting your life.** Besides telling your doctor how it's affecting your energy, the quality of your sleep, and your ability to exercise, describe how it's influencing your mood and well-being, your relationships, and your ability to function at home and at work.

- **Don't give up until you achieve good pain management.** Sometimes it can take a while to find the right combination of approaches and strategies that will ease *your* pain. If you don't feel like you're getting onto the right track with your doctor, ask for a referral to a specialist.

The State of Your Social Life

We are, from our earliest origins, social creatures who are highly influenced by our relationships with others. This isn't just a warm and fuzzy topic. The cold, hard scrutiny of clinical trials has demonstrated that people with loving, supportive relationships are far less vulnerable to chronic diseases and death than those who don't have positive relationships. Simply having friends helps protect our health. People with good social networks tend to be more physically and psychologically resilient, and more optimistic. They're less susceptible to the common cold and less prone to inflammation, and they have more robust immune responses to vaccines. Social support also may have positive effects on the number and behavior of white blood cells and brain wave patterns.

The flip side can be detrimental. Research from Harvard University found that people with chronically higher levels of "social strain" (negative interactions with family members and friends) have abnormal cortisol-release rhythms throughout the day, which places stress on their bodies and minds. (If there are family members in your household with whom you don't get along, that's a problem in its own right. Improving the state of your relationship may be the first order of business, before you can enlist that person's support for the lifestyle changes you're making.)

To elicit the assistance and encouragement you want and need from your family, friends, and colleagues, try the following strategies:

- **Identify the most supportive people in your life.** If you do this well before you need their support, you'll feel better knowing you have people—a whole network, really—to turn to in a pinch.
- **Maintain a spirit of give-and-take.** Sometimes you'll be the one giving support; other times you'll be the one getting it. Make sure it continues to be a two-way street to avoid overburdening your friends and family.
- **Ask for help.** Confide in the people you trust about how you're feeling, and let family and friends help you manage your challenges better. To get the kind of support you really want and need, be specific in telling them how they can best help you.
- **Communicate constructively.** To try to defuse tension from difficult relationships, express yourself directly but tactfully by calmly describing your needs or feelings using statements that begin with *I*, then outline your request for change, action, or support. Don't complain, whine, or hurl accusations.
- **Expand your social circle.** You can do this by volunteering for a cause or charity you believe in, exercising at a gym, joining a hobby club (such as a walking club or a book group), or taking a class.

Each of these factors—sleep, stress management, social support, and pain control—can improve the state of your health on their own. What's more, they can have a cumulative, synergistically positive effect on bolstering your health and well-being. But as you can see, the converse is true as well: Too little good-quality shut-eye, too much stress (or poorly managed stress), too little social support and love, and too much pain can take a toll on your physical and emotional health. If you're batting 0 for 4, the toll is even greater.

Achieving the Right Ripple Effect

Reversing a downward health trajectory often begins with one well-prioritized move in the opposite direction. If the erosion of health is a degenerating spiral, then reclaiming health requires ascending the spiral. Each step you climb puts you in a better position to climb the next one, and it brings you closer to the luminous prize at the top: vitality. Once you begin climbing, you'll likely find that the skills you need to take each step enhance each other, build upon each other, and create a positive synergy that leads to their positive reinforcement of each other. In other words, each skill you acquire makes you better at the next, and the next, and so on. When you reach the pinnacle of that spiral (your optimum vitality), you'll likely gain more years in your life and better quality life in your years.

The best way to set that positive chain reaction into motion is to find your natural entry point for the Skill Spiral, a customizable plan that maps out a clear course for you to develop specific health-promoting skills. Think of it as the antidote to circling the drain: By devising a sequential process of acquiring one health-promoting skill, then another, and another, you'll be able to ascend the spiral to better health. Before you can figure out how to do that, you'll want to prioritize the skills you want to develop so you can gain traction and make more rapid progress on your journey to a healthier you.

Using the boxes that follow in the Disease-Proofing Profiler will help you figure out the optimal sequence of steps for getting the skillpower you need. Once you have identified that sequence, imagine placing those priorities (and the skills that come with them) on the steps that ascend your personal Skill Spiral. As you address those priorities and build those skills one by one, you'll start to rise higher toward your goal of greater vitality and better health. The profiler has four domains: *forest, family and friends, feet*, and *fork*. Review the contents of the boxes on each domain, one at a time, to decide if you need to address skills within that domain. If so, rank the challenges in order of their priority for you, with 1 representing the highest priority. Priority status is subjective; it should be based on your sense about which items are most challenging or important for you personally. You may want to think in terms of "I'm sure I could do *that*, if only I could do *this* . . ." which would make *this* a higher priority than *that*. Once you have completed your priority lists for all four boxes, you have essentially established your personal route up through the Skill Spiral.

Forest

Forest refers to the big picture, seeing the forest despite the trees so you can get out of the woods and improve your overall health. It's premature to start working on your diet and physical activity if you are burdened by sleep problems, excess stress, or chronic pain. If you have any of the impediments in the "Forest" box, then your Skill Spiral will start there, working through these "big picture" challenges in order of their priority to you, using the guidance provided.

**Table 12.1 The Forest: Addressing the Big
Picture of Your Overall Health**

Situation	Priority	Guidance
Insufficient sleep		Chapter 12
Stress overload		Chapters 5, 12
Chronic pain		Chapter 12
Social isolation		Chapter 12

Family and Friends

Family and friends refers to your household situation. If you have a spouse, significant other, or even roommates, their lifestyle is likely to influence yours, and vice versa. If you have children, they can make eating well and being active easier or harder. In unity, there is strength; without unity, changing your habits can feel like an uphill climb. Your close relationships are a part of your journey to better health, and they need to figure into your formula for skill development. Unless you are truly going it alone, identify your situation in the "Family and Friends" box, and determine your sequence of priorities there, working through them with the guidance provided. If you have Forest steps, the Family and Friends steps will be the second set to add to your Spiral; otherwise, this will be where your staircase begins.

Table 12.2. Family and Friends: Addressing the Key Relationships That Affect Your Daily Routine

Situation	Priority	Guidance
Spouse or significant other		Chapters 7, 8, 9, 10
Children		Chapters 7, 8, 9, 10
Roommates		Chapters 7, 8, 10
Large social network		Chapters 9, 10

Feet

Feet refers to your physical activity pattern, of course, and the impediments that stand between you and fitting fitness (or more of it) in. Identify the main reason(s) it's hard for you to be more active, and work through those in order of their priority to you, using the guidance provided. If you don't have Forest or Family and Friends steps, you'll start here; otherwise, Feet will follow your last set of steps.

Table 12.3. Feet: Addressing Your Physical Activity Pattern

Situation	Priority	Guidance
Lack motivation to exercise		Chapters 2, 10
Difficulty fitting activity in		Chapters 10, 11
Trouble establishing an exercise program		Chapter 10
Get bored with exercise		Chapter 10

Fork

Fork refers to your dietary pattern and the impediments that stand between you and eating better for the rest of your life. Identify the most important barriers to your eating well, and work through them in order of their priority to you, using the guidance provided. This will be the last set of steps in your sequence—or perhaps you are entering the spiral here if the other categories don't pertain to you.

**Table 12.4. Fork: Addressing the Overall
Picture of Your Dietary Issues**

Situation	Priority	Guidance
Lack general nutrition knowledge		Chapter 4
Prefer unhealthy foods		Chapter 6
Have trouble affording nutritious foods		Chapter 7
Lack cooking skills		Chapter 8
Have difficulty eating well on the road		Chapter 9
Can't control eating behavior		Chapter 5

The Skill Spiral

Once you have your priorities set from using the Profiler, you're ready to map out your ascension of the Skill Spiral. At the start of the skill acquisition period, everybody should do the following two things: First, if you are currently not exercising at all, use the guidance in chapter 11 to sneak bouts of physical activity into the nooks and crannies of your day. Second, start to control your food choices by making use of a well-provisioned snack pack that you can take with you when you're away from home (see chapter 9 for suggestions). These two steps are so important because they provide an immediate boost to your sense of control and empowerment, and your self-esteem, which can help you build momentum toward your goals. They allow you to send yourself a message that health is a priority *today*, which can help you make better choices as you continue.

Devote up to two weeks to working through the skills in each domain—if you have things to address in all four areas, that means you'll be taking about eight weeks in total to complete all the steps in your Skill Spiral. If you find that you can't address everything in one area in two weeks, take as long as you need. The important thing is that you're making these changes!

While one circuit through the Skill Spiral is intended to give you the skillpower you need to set you on the course to lasting vitality, there is no reason that building your skillpower needs to end there. It is always possible for us to learn new skills or to get better at ones we already have. Even master carpenters can benefit from learning how to use a new tool. Developing skillpower for better health is like that, too, so remember that you can reformulate and follow your personal Skill Spiral as many times as you want to make the journey.

By completing a circuit of the Spiral, you will have acquired not only a powerful set of skills, but also mastery of the *method* for acquiring skills! You will have hands-on experience in sizing up obstacles that lie in your path and tracking down the information, program, resource, tool, or other source of help you need to get past it. Skillpower really is the combination of *having* a whole set of skills and having the requisite skills for acquiring new skills as you need them. With commitment and the right skillpower, you can almost certainly find a way to rise a considerable distance toward the heights of greater vitality and disease-proofing your future. But there is no helicopter that will swoop in to take you up there. The climb needs to be made one skill-based step at a time.

Keep in mind that the behaviors that prevent chronic disease and premature death should not be substituted for one another; they should coexist harmoniously so they can work in concert and have an additive effect upon one another. Only then can you begin to reap the benefits of the cumulative effect of these interconnected skills. Plus, each thing you do to take care of your health helps you feel more capable, which makes it easier for you to do something else to improve your health, which also helps you feel better about yourself, and so on.

Call it a positive feedback loop, a virtuous cycle, or a beneficial ripple effect—by any name, this investment in your well-being can yield substantial gains. It really does work. In a study involving 170 people who were trying to lose weight, researchers at the University of Pittsburgh School of Nursing found that when participants adhered to a limited fat intake, their sense of self-efficacy (their belief in their ability to succeed) improved, and the higher their self-efficacy became, the greater their weight loss was over the eighteen-month treatment period.

The way toward a healthier future may require taking a step backward to a simpler way of living—to a style of life that involves consuming more foods that come directly from nature and engaging in more movement instead of relying so much on laborsaving devices. In other words, we now have to think about doing the health-promoting things that came naturally in the past. This includes making it a priority to get good-quality sleep and enough of it, to manage stress in healthy ways (through exercise, deep breathing, meditation, and the like), and to nurture our relationships even (or especially) when life is hectic.

Sure, you may encounter some unexpected obstacles along the way.

But one of the most empowering things about acquiring skillpower is that you learn how to acquire the skills you need as you need them. The process becomes familiar, and you'll come to own it. To paraphrase poet Theodore Roethke, you'll learn by going where you have to go. That's the power of skill synergy at its best.

Thirteen

The Levee: Thinking Globally, Acting Locally, Changing the World

Much of this book has focused on using your feet and fork as the master levers of medical destiny, and the idea that they are yours to control. You don't need to keep on waiting for the world to change! You're taking steps to enhance your own health right now.

But it would be nice if the world *did* change, so that better health and weight control moved from the road less traveled (at least by our culture) to a path of much less resistance for us all. The problem is that none of us is directly in charge of all the relevant factors in modern society that promote obesity and chronic disease. But those detrimental influences should be fixed. Yet, as we all know, culture, society, and institutions change slowly and often reluctantly. For now, it's up to us to overcome them through skillpower. Why wait when you don't have to?

While each of us can develop the right skillpower to protect the health of our own bodies, and perhaps the bodies of those we love, only the body politic can change policies, programs, and culture itself so that becoming healthier and controlling our weight are simply the norm. That can happen—it should happen—and each of us can be a part of it.

The Three Musketeers famously gave us the motto "All for one, and one for all!" The notion of working to protect one another's welfare and fight for the greater good is unquestionably noble. Unfortunately, when it comes to promoting public health (a greater good if ever there was one), the reality is that garnering any individual's passion for an anonymous *all* is elusive at best. This is understandable because the *public* is nameless and faceless. So it's hard to keep in mind that "an 80 percent reduction in chronic disease" actually means that heart attacks and cancer won't occur among the people you love and care about when they otherwise would have. If we're going to reform our health-harming, obesity-promoting environment and make it more health-enhancing, there need to be key policy changes that will allow us collectively to create a lifestyle that's conducive to the healthy use of feet and forks.

To consider the ways in which the world should change, it helps to think about building a levee. I like this metaphor for three reasons. First, when it comes to our efforts to eat well and be active every day, to lose and/or control our weight, and to find better health, we are all facing a veritable flood of opposing forces. The flood includes highly processed, energy-dense, nutrient-poor, hyper-palatable, or glow-in-the-dark foods. It includes a constant flow of marketing dollars that encourage us, and our kids, to eat ever more of the very foods that propel us toward obesity and chronic disease. Wave after wave of technological advances give us gadgets and gizmos that do all the things our muscles used to do. Our hectic work schedules leave us little time for attention to health. Our agricultural policies subsidize corn to fatten cows, rather than vegetables and fruits to vitalize people. It's a vast, obesity-promoting, health-compromising flood.

In fact, if we compare this world we've created to the past, this is the reality: Throughout most of human history, calories were relatively scarce and hard to get, and physical activity was unavoidable. Now the opposite is true: Physical activity is relatively scarce and hard to get, and calories are unavoidable. Plus we're surrounded by all the wrong kinds of calories (from highly processed foods with little nutritional value). Houston, we have a problem! If you want to contain a flood and turn the tide, you build a levee. We can achieve it one sandbag at a time. No one sandbag can make a whole levee, and no one program, policy, or tool is the whole solution to our obesity-promoting, disease-favoring world, either. But we can move toward the definitive solution, one step at a time. And, in fact, there is some evidence that we are doing just that. A September 2012 report by the Robert Wood Johnson Foundation indicates that rates of childhood obesity are actually declining slightly in cities throughout the United States where the most efforts are being undertaken to prevent this problem.

Also in 2012, the Institute of Medicine released its report on what it will take to fix the problem of epidemic obesity. The novel elements that figured in the report included a new perspective on the price tag—the opportunity to save or spend over half a trillion dollars on obesity between now and 2030. In the IOM report, entitled "Accelerating Progress in Obesity Prevention: Solving the Weight of the Nation," an expert panel distilled the solution down to these five key points: Integrate physical activity every day in every way; market what matters for a healthy life; make healthy foods and beverages available everywhere; activate employers and health care professionals; and strengthen schools as the heart of health. We need sandbags to address each of these issues.

The levee metaphor serves up a cautionary message for us all about what it actually takes to get the job done. No one little thing is *the* answer. My colleagues and I have published several systematic reviews and meta-analyses of obesity prevention and control. These studies look diligently at the prior research and pool results to reach a conclusion from high altitude. What we've seen is that, despite the challenges, many interventions do show promise in preventing or reversing obesity. But many, many more show promise as part of a larger solution. (Figure 13.1 shows a "causal pathway" for the development of obesity and the chronic diseases that tend to follow in its wake.)

We can work long, hard, and constructively and still see no results at all, because we have just been assembling the various parts of the solution. We won't really see results until we put everything together, just as a flood is contained only when an adequate levee is fully built.

What are the components (the sandbags) of this anti-obesity, prohealth solution? For starters, we could make everyone a nutrition expert by putting an objective, evidence-based, at-a-glance measure of overall nutritional quality on display everywhere that people and food come together—and thus close every loophole to marketing distortions. We can

Figure 13.1: An Ecological Model of Diet, Physical Activity, and Obesity

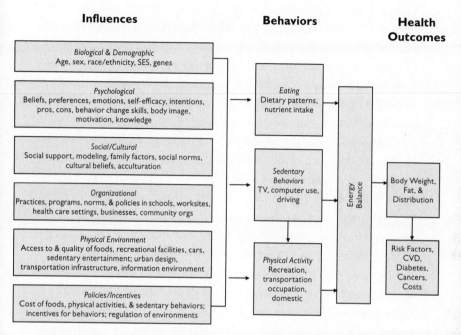

Developed for the NHLBI Workshop on Predictors of Obesity, Weight Gain, Diet, and Physical Activity: August 4–5, 2004, Bethesda MD

change what restaurants and supermarkets serve by changing what we choose. That's the very purpose of the NuVal System described earlier, but thus far, only a small portion of the total population has access to NuVal Scores or any comparable system. We could build from there and attach a system of financial incentives so that the more nutritious the food, the less it costs. The incentives would provide an opportunity for savings to be paid by the entities that currently pay the costs of disease care: insurance companies, large employers, and the federal government. The cost of subsidizing cabbage (in the produce aisle) is trivial compared to the cost of CABG (coronary artery bypass grafting) in the operating room, according to some of the world's leading health economists. Setting incentives for people to make healthful choices could save us a lot of money, individually and as a nation. Everyone can win.

We could create and encourage access to physical activity programs that embrace the principle of sound mind, sound body and that honor personal preferences for different kinds of exercise. Every school could support this without giving up time for reading, writing, or arithmetic. (That's what the free ABC for Fitness program is for.) Similarly, every worksite and church could provide opportunities for movement, such as the free ABE for Fitness program, to help adults fit in bouts of physical activity anywhere, anytime. Instant Recess, a program developed by Dr. Toni Yancey of UCLA, is tailor-made to get groups, such as church congregations, up and moving for ten minutes at a time. We can alter the workplace by getting together with like-minded coworkers, and expressing a collective opinion to management about bringing in healthier foods and encouraging physical activity.

Little by little, we could improve our built environments so that every neighborhood and town was designed to make physical activity a regular part of daily life. As neighborhoods grow, evolve, or begin, we should restore the options for the person-powered transportation (a.k.a. active transportation) we once had. The White House Task Force on Childhood Obesity has set a goal of increasing walking and biking to school by 50 percent in the next five years—that's a goal every family with a child can help the nation realize, even if it means driving part of the way, parking the car, and walking the rest. Businesses also could provide and reward bike-to-work practices, which would contribute to the health of people and the environment alike.

While doing all that you can right now to put *your* feet to good use, you can do everybody else's feet a favor by encouraging policy makers to advance legislation and funding that will improve the "walkability" of neighborhoods. In addition, we should urge them to work to create new walking trails, bike lanes, parks, and open spaces, so that there are more opportunities and resources for residents to safely and easily engage in walking, biking, and other ways of being physically active. Research has found that adults who live in highly walkable neighborhoods do more moderate and vigorous physical activity, *and* they're less likely to be overweight than adults who live in neighborhoods that aren't so walkable.

In the meantime, many schools and businesses could become sources of real, healthy food by getting involved in the edible garden movement. Our schools could teach children and their parents the skills that are required to identify and choose more nutritious foods (perhaps using the Nutrition Detectives program). Cafeterias could be designed to gently encourage better choices. A nationwide survey found that parents seek ways to combat childhood obesity more often from schools than they do from health care providers and government agencies. To some extent, this makes sense, given that no other institution has as much continuous and intensive contact with children. But there really needs to be a nationwide mandate to have schools help combat obesity by offering more frequent physical education classes and recess, healthy school meals and snacks, health and nutrition education, and good-quality health services. Until that happens, broach the subject at school open houses, PTA meetings, and parent-teacher conferences. To help with the cost of such measures, businesses could adopt schools (as they now adopt highways) to provide the resources required for state-of-the-art health-promotion programming.

There is evidence that young children gain more weight over the summer, when they're away from the disciplined structure of school, than they do during the academic year. So even good school policies will not be enough; we need health-promoting routines to follow kids home, too. For kids with more extreme needs, we should make more resources available. Imagine a boarding school where obese kids get a fully accredited semester of high school, lose 50 to 100 pounds, escape the bullying that so often adds insult to the injury of poor health, and recover their self-esteem. This actually exists, at the MindStream Academy in South Carolina, where I serve as medical adviser. What we need now is for insurers to cover a life-changing semester at this kind of school, just as they cover the costs of bariatric surgery. The benefits of developing healthy skillpower can be paid forward, whereas a rewiring of the gastrointestinal tract can't be.

Similarly, more family-friendly weight-management programs that are just as focused on improving health as on losing weight should be developed—and insurers should cover participation in these. After all, insurance plans already cover the costs of dealing with the poor health that results when weight gets out of control. Yet the skills for weight management and healthy living are largely neglected by insurance policies.

On the food front, the marketing of foods to children can, and should, be regulated—not because we want the government to tell us what to have for breakfast, but because pitting high-paid executives on Madison Avenue against your six-year-old just isn't fair! There's no reason for highly trained and very clever adults to profit from talking young children into doing things that are likely to make them chronically ill. It is, in fact, unconscionable. Many other countries have already reached this very reasonable conclusion. We should also shift government subsidies and marketing regulations from foods with the longest shelf lives to foods that extend the shelf lives of the people who are eating them.

And while we're at it, we could eradicate tobacco use, which remains a hugely important health influence at the societal level. For far too long already this pernicious scourge has robbed people of the good health and longevity they might otherwise have enjoyed. Those currently addicted to tobacco should need a physician's authorization to get it, and they should also receive every form of assistance modern science can offer to help them quit. But the substance, and any marketing of it, should be banned for all others. No young person should ever again be seduced into smoking.

We could do all this, and more, until the 80 percent of all chronic diseases that can be eliminated are actually eliminated, and not just for those of us willing to take disease-proofing into our own hands. This is what building the levee would look like. Chronic health could replace chronic disease, and the burden of making it happen wouldn't rest with you or me but with all of us. It truly does take a village to build a healthier environment.

Is all this realistic? Certainly not right away, which is why most of this book is devoted to the action you can take right away to defend your health in spite of it all. But of course, we can change policy by changing the priorities that influence how we vote. Mayors and governors are obligated to care about the things voters care about, and these officials are in turn responsible for appointing urban planners and the people who run zoning and planning, parks and recreation. As the famous saying goes, the best way to predict the future is to create it! Health-promoting changes in our culture and environment will certainly never happen if we don't envision them.

Throughout this book, we have made the case that we can change our lifestyle habits. But we can also control our culture, since, collectively, we created it in the first place. We could change our culture to make health a prevailing priority—not in one fell swoop, but in lots of small steps that would add up over time. Ultimately, we, as a society and as individuals, can change our ways and protect the health of our children and grandchildren by promoting an environment that honors feet, forks, and fingers as the tools that can change our medical future. This would be a welcome relief from relying so heavily on stethoscopes, scalpels, and statins in the aftermath of unnecessary crises. What we need to do is create the path of least resistance to eating well and being active. As the famous cultural anthropologist Margaret Mead told us, "Never doubt that a small group of thoughtful and committed citizens can change the world. Indeed, it is the only thing that ever has." So while taking personal action, let's also be part of that group of thoughtful and committed citizens—and change the world for the better, so that health lies along that path of lesser resistance for everyone.

At a meeting in Montreal a couple of years ago, I was fortunate to meet the husband-and-wife team who started a business called Real Food for Real Kids (www.rfrk.com) in Toronto. The idea was born when this couple couldn't find a day-care center that served fresh, tasty, wholesome lunches and snacks when they needed one for their children. So they started making healthy, wholesome foods for their son to take to day care. Then, upon request, they began providing food for the whole day care, then for a dozen day-care centers in their area. Last I heard, they were feeding nearly six thousand children every day with wholesome, homemade foods—using organic ingredients such as whole grains, legumes, colorful vegetables, fresh fruit, and lean meats, poultry, or fish—while supporting local farmers who were using sustainable methods. This is good for the land, good for the children, and, as it turns out, a really good business.

When enough of us act locally, we become part of that group of committed citizens who truly can change the world for the better. So consider the possibilities and what you can do to help the process along. And then just imagine bequeathing to your children a future—and a culture—in which disease-proofing ourselves comes naturally, as a regular part of life. If we can imagine it, we can make it happen. If we can predict the future we would like for ourselves and our children, little by little we can work together to create it!

Acknowledgments

I am, as ever, dedicated to the community of scientists who have shown us the potential we have to add years to our lives and better quality life to our years. I don't dare name names for fear of overlooking innumerable others who are just as noteworthy. I acknowledge science itself, and all who propagate it and thereby provide the knowledge that is a prerequisite to power. I am privileged when I can make my own modest contributions to our fund of practical knowledge, and I am indebted to the arduous toil and incremental gains of science, as are we all.

More specifically, I thank Rick Broadhead, who is now as much friend as literary agent, and greatly valued in both roles. I am deeply thankful for the careful editing provided by Christina Rodriguez and Caroline Sutton at Penguin, and for their support of this effort. I thank them as well for that unique brand of solicitous discipline authors tend to need to turn a mad jumble of ideas into an actual book.

I thank my wife, Catherine, and my children, for graciously accommodating the many hours during which this book had my attention and they did not. Stacey and I are also grateful to Catherine for the wonderful recipes we offer in *Disease-Proof*. Catherine's culinary talent has always enabled the Katz family to love food that loves us back. By sharing her recipes here, we hope to pay that opportunity forward to many other families.

And most of all, I thank my coauthor, Stacey Colino, for long and uncomplaining hours of hard work, good cheer, great insight, apparent immunity to writer's block, and unfailing professionalism. I could not imagine a better partner, and am proud to share this product of long labors with her.

Daily Food Diary

Use the following chart to help you assess what you're eating, how much, and why. It's especially helpful in identifying emotional reasons for eating—so you can discover what specific *need* is actually being fed.

Meal/ Snack	Descriptors	Day of the Week/ Date: Workday? Y/N
BREAKFAST	What and how much	
	When and where	
	Why	
A.M. SNACK(S)	What and how much	
	When and where	
	Why	
LUNCH	What and how much	
	When and where	
	Why	

(continued)

Meal/ Snack	Descriptors	Day of the Week/ Date: Workday? Y/N
P.M. SNACK(S)	What and how much	
	When and where	
	Why	
DINNER	What and how much	
	When and where	
	Why	
EVENING SNACK(S)	What and how much	
	When and where	
	Why	
OTHER (ALCOHOL, BEVERAGES)	What and how much	
	When and where	
	Why	

NuVal® Scores*

The NuVal® Nutritional Scoring System ranks foods from different categories on a scale from 1 to 100—the higher the number, the more nutritious the food is. The system, which allows you to compare the overall nutritional quality of one product to another, has been used to score well over 100,000 foods and is available in approximately 1,700 supermarkets across the country. (To find one near you, visit www.nuval.com.) If you have access to the system, use it; if you don't, here's a look at the range of scores, displayed from high to low, to give you a sense of the extent to which foods within the same category can vary in nutritional value.

BREAD (Score range displayed: 14–50)	NuVal® Score (1–100)
Nature's Own Double Fiber Wheat Bread	50
Pepperidge Farm Whole Grain Bread 15 Grain Hearty Texture	48
Nature's Own 100% Whole Grain Bread	45
Wonder Special Recipe Bread 100% Whole Wheat Smart White Bread	44

(continued)

*Disclaimer: The scores are based on information on the packaging and are subject to change as packaging is updated.

BREAD	NuVal® Score (1–100)
Sara Lee 100% Multi-Grain Bread	40
Arnold Country Whole Grain White Bread	39
Pepperidge Farm Stone Ground 100% Whole Wheat Bread	38
Vermont Bread Company Yoga Bread	36
Sunbeam Lite Bread Wheat	35
Sara Lee 100% Whole Wheat Bakery Bread	34
Freihofer's Family 100% Whole Wheat Bread	34
Wonder Whole Grain White Bread	31
Arnold Whole Grains Health Nut Bread	30
Home Pride Whole Grains 100% Whole Wheat Bread	29
Pepperidge Farm Oatmeal Bread	28
Wonder Calcium Fortified Enriched Bread	28
Sara Lee Jewish Rye Bakery Bread	27
Freihofer's Split Top Wheat Bread	26
Pepperidge Farm Deli Swirl Rye & Pump Bread	25
Arnold Brick Oven Enriched Premium White Bread	25
Arnold Hearth Stone Bread Wheat	25
Pepperidge Farm Italian Bread with Sesame Seeds	24
Arnold Jewish Rye Bread Seedless	24
Nature's Own Honey Wheat Enriched Bread	23
Pepperidge Farm Simply Natural Honey Oat Bread	23
Pepperidge Farm Farmhouse Hearty Sliced Bread, Oatmeal	18
Home Pride Butter Top Enriched White Bread	14

(continued)

COOKIES (Score range displayed: 1–33)	NuVal® Score (1–100)
Kashi Oatmeal Raisin Flax Soft-Baked Cookies	33
Nabisco Newtons Fruit Thins Crispy Cookies, Blueberry Brown Sugar	27
Quaker Crunchy Oat Granola Cookies, Apple & Cinnamon	26
Voortman Oatmeal Cranberry Flaxseed Omega 3 Cookies	26
Annie's Homegrown Bunny Grahams Honey Whole Grain Graham Snacks	25
Barbara's Snackimals Animal Cookies, Peanut Butter	24
Kashi TLC Oatmeal Dark Chocolate Soft-Baked Cookies	23
Nabisco 100 Cal Chips Ahoy Thin Crisps Baked Chocolate Chip Snacks	21
Quaker Soft Baked Oatmeal Cookies, Cranberry & Yogurt	20
Nabisco Teddy Grahams Graham Snacks, Chocolatey Chip	16
Keebler Vanilla Wafers	16
Keebler Gripz Mighty Tiny Chocolate Chip Cookies, Chips Deluxe Cookies	15
Weight Watchers Chocolate Chip Cookies	14
Nabisco Newtons Original Fig Chewy Cookies	13
Nabisco Chips Ahoy! Original Cookies	13
Murray Sugar Free Cookies, Chocolate Chip	12
Keebler Cinnamon Roll Cookies, Caramel Pecan	10
Nabisco Lorna Doone Shortbread Cookies	9
Nabisco Reduced Fat Oreo Chocolate Sandwich Cookies	9

(continued)

COOKIES	NuVal® Score (1–100)
Pepperidge Farm Milano Melts Dark Classic Crème Crispy Cookies	9
Back to Nature California Lemon Cookies	8
Nabisco SnackWell's Fudge Drizzled Chocolate Chip Cookies	7
Grandma's Homestyle Oatmeal Raisin Cookies	7
Nabisco Nilla Wafers	6
Keebler Fudge Stripes Cookies Original	5
Nabisco Double Stuf Oreo Chocolate Sandwich Cookies	4
Keebler Soft Batch Cookies, Chocolate Chip	3
Pepperidge Farm Milano Distinctive Cookies	2
Archway Homestyle Cookies Iced Circus Animals	1

CRACKERS (Score range displayed: 4–63)	NuVal® Score (1–100)
Streit's Unsalted Matzos	63
Go Raw Organic Sunflower Flax Snax	60
Kashi Heart to Heart Original Whole Grain Crackers	38
Nabisco Baked 100% Whole Grain Wheat Triscuit Crackers	38
Kellogg's All-Bran Crackers Multi-Grain Bite-Size Baked Snacks	37
Nabisco Wheat Thins Fiber Selects Garden Vegetable Crackers	34
Nabisco Triscuit Reduced Fat Baked Whole Grain Wheat Crackers	32
Back to Nature 100% Natural Harvest Whole Wheats Crackers	30

(continued)

CRACKERS	NuVal® Score (1–100)
Pepperidge Farm Harvest Wheat Distinctive Crackers	29
Keebler Town House Light Buttery Crackers, Wheat	28
Nabisco Wheat Thins Reduced Fat Snacks	28
Keebler Club Crackers, Multi-Grain	27
Kellogg's Special K Cracker Chips Baked Snacks, Sea Salt	27
Back to Nature 100% Natural Spinach & Roasted Garlic Crackers	26
Pepperidge Farm Goldfish Baked Snack Crackers	25
Pepperidge Farm Baked Naturals Cracker Chips, Simply Potato	24
Sunshine Cheez-It Baked Snack Crackers Reduced Fat	23
Back to Nature 100% Natural Sunflower Basil Crackers	22
Pepperidge Farm Goldfish Baked Snack Crackers, Pretzel	18
Nabisco Ritz Whole Wheat Crackers	13
Nabisco Ritz Reduced Fat Crackers	12
Nabisco Unsalted Tops Premium Saltine Crackers	11
Carr's Whole Wheat Crackers	10
Pepperidge Farm Golden Butter Distinctive Crackers	9
Blue Diamond Hazelnut Nut-Thins Nut & Rice Cracker Snacks	8
Nabisco Original Topped with Sea Salt Premium Saltine Crackers	7
Annie's Homegrown Organic Bunny Classics Cheddar Crackers	6
Back to Nature Gluten Free White Cheddar Rice Thin Crackers	4

(continued)

CEREALS (Score range displayed: 8–91)	NuVal® Score (1–100)
Bear River Valley Toasted Tumble All Natural Whole Grain Wheat Cereal	91
Kashi 7 Whole Grain Puffs	91
Post Shredded Wheat Spoon Size Original Cereal	91
Nature's Path Organic Corn Puffs Cereal	87
General Mills Fiber One Original Bran Cereal	53
Kellogg's All-Bran Original Cereal	47
Kashi Autumn Wheat Organic Whole Wheat Biscuits	44
Kind Cinnamon Oat Clusters with Flax Seeds	42
Natural Ovens Bakery Great Granola Cereal	39
Nature's Path Organic Hemp Plus Granola Cereal	39
General Mills Cheerios Toasted Whole Grain Oat Cereal	37
Kashi Heart to Heart Warm Cinnamon Oat Cereal	36
Kellogg's Frosted Original Mini-Wheats Bite Size Cereal	33
General Mills Total Crunchy Whole Grain Wheat Flakes	31
Kashi GoLean Crisp! Multigrain Cluster Cereal, Toasted Berry Crumble	30
Barbara's Original Puffins Cereal	29
General Mills Wheaties	28
Kellogg's Raisin Bran	27
Kellogg's Special K Red Berries Cereal	25
Quaker Life Cereal	25
Kellogg's Cracklin' Oat Bran Cereal	23
Kellogg's Special K Original Lightly Toasted Rice Cereal	20

(continued)

CEREALS	NuVal® Score (1–100)
Cascadian Farm Organic Oats and Honey Granola	20
Post Waffle Crisp Sweetened Multi-Grain Cereal	14
Kellogg's Smorz Crunchy Graham Cereal	11
Cap'n Crunch Sweetened Corn & Oat Cereal	10
Kellogg's Rice Krispies Treats Cereal	8

JUICES (Score range displayed: 1–82)	NuVal® Score (1–100)
Lakewood Organic Fresh Pressed Pure Cranberry 100% Juice	82
Red Gold No Salt Added 100% Tomato Juice from Concentrate	82
Tropicana No Pulp Calcium + Vitamin D Trop 50 Orange Juice Beverage	81
Lakewood Organic Fresh Pressed Pure Carrot 100% Juice	76
Lakewood Organic Fresh Blends Mango 100% Juice Blend	67
Campbell's V8 Low Sodium Original 100% Vegetable Juice	53
Apple & Eve Fruitables Vegetable Juice Beverage, Fruit Punch	51
Florida's Natural Premium 100% Pasteurized Orange Juice, with Calcium & Vitamin D	49
Tropicana Pure Premium 100% Orange Juice with Calcium & Vitamin D	49
Florida's Natural Premium 100% Pasteurized Grapefruit Juice with Calcium	47

(continued)

JUICES	NuVal® Score (1–100)
Simply Orange 100% Pure Squeezed Pasteurized Orange Juice with Calcium & Vitamin D, Pulp Free	47
Naked Mighty Mango 100% Juice Smoothie	44
Red Gold Vegetable Juice from Concentrate	43
Dole Pineapple Juice 100% Juice Fortified with Vitamins A, C & E	41
Lakewood Organic Fresh Pressed Blueberry 100% Juice Blend	41
Campbell's V8 Original 100% Vegetable Juice	40
Mott's Garden Blend 100% Vegetable Juice	38
Lakewood Organic Pomegranate 100% Juice Blend	37
R.W. Knudsen Family Very Veggie 100% Vegetable Juice Blend	36
Del Monte Pineapple Juice from Concentrate 100% Juice	34
Minute Maid Premium Heart Wise 100% Orange Juice	32
Kraft Capri Sun Super V Fruit & Vegetable Juice Drink	30
Old Orchard Healthy Balance Pomegranate Reduced Sugar Juice Cocktail Blend	29
Sunsweet Plum Smart Light Juice Cocktail	28
Jumex Peach Nectar	26
Welch's 100% Grape Juice No Sugar Added	25
Mott's Plus Light Apple Juice Beverage	22
Sunsweet 100% Juice Plum Smart Juice	22
Apple & Eve 100% Juice White Grape Raspberry Flavored Blend	18
Snapple Fruit Punch 100% Juice	16

(continued)

JUICES	NuVal® Score (1–100)
Nestlé Juicy Juice Fruitifuls All Natural Apple Quench Flavored Juice Beverage	13
Nestlé Juicy Juice All Natural 100% Juice, Orange Tangerine	11
Goya Pear Nectar	7
Bolthouse Farms Mango Lemonade Juice Beverage	6
Kraft Capri Sun Wakeup Orange Flavored Juice Drink Blend	4
Arizona Original Brand Watermelon Fruit Juice Cocktail	3
Hawaiian Punch Juice Drink, Fruit Juicy Red	3
Sunny D Tangy Original Orange Flavored Citrus Punch	3
Snapple Peach Mangosteen Juice Drink	2
Welch's Concord Grape Fruit Juice Cocktail	2
Minute Maid Premium Fruit Punch Juice Blend	1
Simply Lemonade	1

PASTA SAUCES (Score range displayed: 9–92)	NuVal® Score (1–100)
Francesco Rinaldi Traditional (No Salt Added) Pasta Sauce	82
Rao's Homemade Puttanesca—Tomatoes, Capers, Olives & Anchovies	73
Capa Di Roma Marinara	71
Davinci Italian Style Clam Sauce Red	67
Francesco Rinaldi Healthy Garden Vegetable	65
Rao's Homemade Roasted Eggplant Siciliana Sauce	63
Organicville Organic Pasta Sauce, Mushroom	58

(continued)

PASTA SAUCES	NuVal® Score (1–100)
World Classics Trading Company Aromatic Tomato Basil	56
Emeril's All Natural Authentic Recipe Roasted Red Pepper Pasta Sauce	55
Muir Glen Organic Fire Roasted Tomato Organic Pasta Sauce	54
Ragu Old World Style Marinara Smooth Pasta Sauce	53
Newman's Own Marinara Pasta Sauce Made with Extra Virgin Olive Oil	52
Emeril's All Natural Authentic Recipe Home Style Marinara Pasta Sauce	51
Hunt's Premium Traditional	51
Barilla Basilico, Tomato & Basil	50
Bertolli Organic Traditional Tomato & Basil	49
Buitoni Marinara	48
Prego Heart Smart Italian Sauce, Roasted Red Pepper & Garlic	47
Hunt's Pasta Sauce Premium Chunky Vegetable	46
Bertolli Organic, Olive Oil, Basil & Garlic	45
Prego Heart Smart Traditional Italian Sauce	44
Classico Traditional Favorites, Tomato & Basil	43
Essential Everyday Garden Vegetable	42
Bertolli Vidalia Onion with Roasted Garlic Sauce Made with 100% Bertolli Olive Oil	41
Prego Italian Sauce, Fresh Mushroom	39

(continued)

PASTA SAUCES	NuVal® Score (1–100)
Prego Light Smart Traditional Italian Sauce	38
Olde Cape Cod White Clam Sauce With Olive Oil	36
Del Monte Quality Tomato Sauce	34
Ragu Tomato & Basil Light Pasta Sauce	32
Lidia's Artichoke Marinara	30
Newman's Own Made with Extra Virgin Olive Oil, Italian Sausage & Peppers	30
Wolfgang Puck Four Cheese 100% Natural Sauce, Mascarpone, Parmigiano, Ricotta & Asiago	29
Mom's Original Fresh Basil Pasta Sauce, Extra Virgin Olive Oil Artichoke Heart & Asiago Cheese	28
Francesco Rinaldi Meat Flavored Traditional	27
Rao's Homemade Sensitive Formula Marinara	27
Pasta Prima 100% Natural Marinara	26
Pastene Italian Style White Clam Sauce	26
Victoria The Original Four Cheese Pasta Sauce Made with Italian Tomatoes	24
Ragu Cheesy Classic Alfredo Sauce Made with Real Cheese	23
Bertolli Mushroom Alfredo with Portobello Mushrooms Sauce	22
Red Gold Premium Tomatoes	16
Ragu Cheesy Made with Real Cheese Light Parmesan Alfredo	13
Classico Di Parma Signature Recipes, Four Cheese Alfredo	11
Buitoni Alfredo Sauce All Natural	9

(continued)

SALAD DRESSINGS (Score range displayed: 1–13)	NuVal® Score (1–100)
Wish-Bone Light Deluxe French	13
Annie's Naturals Lite Raspberry Vinaigrette	12
Wish-Bone Balsamic Vinaigrette	11
Ken's Steak House Lite Thousand Island	10
Kraft Zesty Italian Anything	10
Maple Grove Farms of Vermont Fat Free Greek	9
Newman's Own Lite Raspberry & Walnut	9
Hidden Valley Farmhouse Originals Dijon Mustard Vinaigrette	8
Newman's Own Lite Honey Mustard	7
Kraft Strawberry Balsamic Vinaigrette	6
Marzetti Simply Dressed Vinaigrette, Strawberry Poppyseed	6
Ken's Steak House Balsamic Vinaigrette	4
Hidden Valley The Original Ranch Old-Fashioned Buttermilk Dressing	3
Kraft Free Zesty Italian Fat Free	2
Maple Grove Farms of Vermont Fat Free Vidalia Onion	1

SALTY SNACKS (Score range displayed: 1–59)	NuVal® Score (1–100)
La Favorita Tortilla Chips, Pinto Bean Lightly Salted	59
Beanfields Bean & Rice Chips, Naturally Unsalted	46
Food Should Taste Good Multigrain Tortilla Chips	43
Mary's Gone Crackers Sticks & Twigs, Chipotle Tomato Light'n Crunchy Pretzel-Snack	40

(continued)

SALTY SNACKS	NuVal® Score (1–100)
Way Better Snacks Simply Sprouted Simply Beyond Black Bean Tortilla Chips	37
Beanfields Bean & Rice Chips, Sea Salt	35
Beanitos Black Bean Chips Chipotle BBQ	32
Food Should Taste Good Brand Original Sweet Potato Chips	31
Cape Cod Kettle Cooked Potato Chips, 40% Reduced Fat	30
Dutch Gourmet Thick Cut Premium Potato Chips, Sea Salt	30
Terra Exotic Vegetable Chips, Mediterranean	30
Kashi Garlic Pesto Pita Crisps	29
Cedar's Baked All Natural Wheat Pita Chips	28
General Mills Simply Chex Cheddar Snacks	28
Cape Cod Kettle Cooked Potato Chips, Original	27
Popchips All Natural Nacho Cheese Tortilla Chips	27
Mission Organics Multigrain Tortilla Chips	26
Smartfood Selects Garlic Tomato Basil Hummus Popped Chips	26
Frito Lay Doritos Cool Ranch Reduced Fat Flavored Tortilla Chips	25
Frito Lay Sun Chips Original Multigrain Snacks	25
Frito Lay Doritos Cool Ranch Flavored Tortilla Chips	24
Rold Gold Pretzels, Sourdough	23
Stacy's Simply Naked Nothing But Sea Salt Pita Chips	19
Kraft Corn Nuts Original Crunchy Corn Snack	16
Frito Lay Lay's Kettle Cooked Original Potato Chips	15

(continued)

SALTY SNACKS	NuVal® Score (1–100)
Frito Lay Fritos Brand Bar-B-Q Flavored Corn Chips	14
Snyder's of Hanover Pretzel Chips Original	12
Frito Lay Lay's Classic Potato Chips	11
General Mills Chex Mix The Original Brand Snack Traditional	7
Rold Gold Pretzels Tiny Twists, Cheddar	7
Mission Organics Multigrain All Natural Tortilla Chips	5
New York Style Original Roasted Garlic Bagel Crisps	5
Pringles Potato Crisps Snack Stacks! The Original	4
Utz Salt'n Vinegar Artificially Flavored Potato Chips	4
Lay's Stax Original Potato Crisps	3
General Mills Bugles Original Corn Snacks	2
Wise Onion Flavored Rings Onion Flavored Snacks	1

YOGURT (Score range displayed: 14–96)	NuVal® Score (1–100)
Dannon All Natural Plain Nonfat Yogurt	96
Yoplait Greek 0% Fat Plain Yogurt	96
Fage Total Nonfat Greek Strained Yogurt	93
Dannon Oikos Greek Nonfat Yogurt, Plain	91
Weight Watchers Berries 'n Cream Nonfat Yogurt	88
Dannon Light & Fit Strawberry Banana Nonfat Yogurt	82
La Yogurt Strawberry Probiotic Blended Nonfat Yogurt	82
Yoplait Light Fat Free Very Vanilla Yogurt	82

(continued)

YOGURT	NuVal® Score (1–100)
Dannon Light & Fit Greek Nonfat Yogurt	57
Chobani Greek Yogurt Flip, Strawberry Sunrise Non-Fat Yogurt with Honey Oats	51
Almond Dream Almond Non-Dairy Yogurt, Coconut Low Fat	49
WholeSoy & Co. Blueberry Soy Yogurt	48
Silk Live! Soy Yogurt, Vanilla	44
Dannon Oikos Greek Strawberry Fruit on the Bottom Nonfat Yogurt	43
Yoplait Greek Blueberry Fruit on the Bottom Fat Free Yogurt	42
Stonyfield Oikos Organic Greek Nonfat Yogurt, Vanilla	41
Dannon All Natural Plain Lowfat Yogurt	40
Fage Total 0% Strawberry Nonfat Greek Strained Yogurt	29
Yoplait Original French Vanilla Flavored Low Fat Yogurt	28
Dannon Activia Selects Parfait Mixed Berry Lowfat Yogurt with Granola Topping	27
Dannon Oikos Traditional Greek Yogurt, Strawberry	27
Yoplait Whips! Peaches 'n Cream Flavored Lowfat Yogurt Mousse	26
Chobani 2% Greek Yogurt Mango Low-Fat Blended Fruit Yogurt	25
The Greek Gods Fig Greek Yogurt Style, Fig On Bottom	24
Brown Cow Blueberry on the Bottom Cream Top Yogurt	23
Dannon Fruit on The Bottom Lowfat Yogurt, Strawberry Banana	23
Müller FrütUp Quaker Very Cherry Lowfat Yogurt with Fruit Mousse	18
Breyers Lowfat Yogurt with Chocolate Flavored Chips	14

(continued)

PRODUCE (Score range displayed: 78–100)	NuVal® Score (1–100)
Asparagus	100
Broccoli	100
Blueberries	100
Green beans	100
Kiwi	100
Oranges	100
Romaine lettuce	100
Spinach	100
Strawberries	100
Carrots	99
Grapefruit (ruby red/pink)	99
Kale	99
Peaches	99
Pineapple	99
Plum	99
Zucchini squash	99
Apples	96
Pears	96
Sweet Potato	96
Tomatoes (red)	96
Mango (red)	93
Potato	93
Bananas (yellow)	91
Corn	91

(continued)

PRODUCE	NuVal® Score (1–100)
Grapes	91
Raspberries (red)	91
Avocados (green)	89
Iceberg lettuce	82
Passion fruit (purple)	78

MEAT/SEAFOOD (Score range displayed: 7–87)	NuVal® Score (1–100)
Atlantic salmon fillet	87
Clams (raw)	82
Snapper	82
Tilapia	82
Shrimp	75
Trout	74
Oyster	66
Haddock	64
Crab (Alaskan King, blue, Dungeness, and snow)	57
Bay scallops	51
Turkey breast (skinless)	48
Chicken breast (skinless)	39
Lobster	36
Pork tenderloin	35

(continued)

MEAT/SEAFOOD	NuVal® Score (1–100)
Beef flank	34
Ground turkey, lean (7% fat)	33
Ground sirloin (90% lean/10% fat)	30
Sirloin beef steak	30
Pork loin chops	28
Ham	27
Porterhouse steak	27
Chuck beef roast	26
Ground beef (70% lean/30% fat)	24
Hormel Smoked Deli Turkey	24
Pork baby back ribs	24
Short beef ribs	24
Butterball Bologna	12
Nathan's Famous The Original Beef Frank	8
Oscar Mayer Naturally Hardwood Smoked Bacon	7

Resources

As you journey along the path to better health, look to these resources to make the trip a bit easier.

FOR YOUR FEET

ABC for Fitness Program (for kids): www.turnthetidefoundation.org/AbcFitness.aspx

ABE for Fitness Program (for adults): www.abeforfitness.com

Instant Recess (a program to get people in workplaces and other groups moving): www.toniyancey.com/IRResources.html

FOR YOUR FINGERS

American Cancer Society (information about the dangers of tobacco and how to quit smoking): www.cancer.org/healthy/stayawayfromtobacco/index

American Heart Association (information about smoking and heart disease): www.heart.org/HEARTORG

American Lung Association (information about how to stop smoking): www.lung.org/stop-smoking

FOR YOUR FORKS

Academy of Nutrition and Dietetics (formerly the American Dietetic Association, for basic nutrition information): www.eatright.org

Food and Drug Administration (information on understanding the Nutrition Facts panel): www.fda.gov/food/ResourcesForYou/Consumers/NFLPM/ucm274593.htm

Healthy Dining Finder (a guide to healthy restaurant options): www.healthydiningfinder.com

Nutrition Detectives: www.davidkatzmd.com/nutritiondetectives.aspx

NuVal Nutritional Scoring System (for use in supermarkets): www.nuval.com

USDA My Plate (which illustrates how to create a healthy plate): www.choosemyplate.gov

Selected Bibliography

Akesson, A., C. Weismayer, P. K. Newby, and A. Wolk. "Combined Effect of Low-Risk Dietary and Lifestyle Behaviors in Primary Prevention of Myocardial Infarction in Women." *Archives of Internal Medicine* 167, no. 19 (October 22, 2007): 2122–27.

Aldana, S. G., R. L. Greenlaw, A. Salberg, H. A. Diehl, R. M. Merrill, C. Thomas, and S. Ohmine. "The Behavioral and Clinical Effects of Therapeutic Lifestyle Change on Middle-Aged Adults." *Preventing Chronic Disease* 3, no. 1 (January 2006): A05.

American Psychological Association. "What Americans Think of Willpower: A Survey of Perceptions of Willpower and Its Role in Achieving Lifestyle and Behavior-Change Goals." 2012. www.apa.org/helpcenter /stress-willpower.pdf (accessed 3/20/2013).

Anderson, L. M., T. A. Quinn, K. Glanz, G. Ramirez, L. C. Kahwati, D. B. Johnson, L. R. Buchanan, W. R. Archer, S. Chattopadhyay, G. P. Kalra, and D. L. Katz. "The Effectiveness of Worksite Nutrition and Physical Activity Interventions for Controlling Employee Overweight and Obesity: A Systematic Review." *American Journal of Preventive Medicine* 37, no. 4 (October 2009): 340–57. Erratum in: *American Journal of Preventive Medicine* 39, no. 1 (July 2010): 104.

Annesi, J. J. "Self-Regulatory Skills Usage Strengthens the Relations of Self-Efficacy for Improved Eating, Exercise, and Weight in the Severely Obese: Toward an Exploratory Model." *Behavioral Medicine* 37, no. 3 (July 2011): 71–76.

Babyak, M., J. A. Blumenthal, S. Herman, P. Khatri, M. Doraiswamy, K. Moore, W. E. Craighead, T. T. Baldewicz, and K. R. Krishnan. "Exercise

Treatment for Major Depression: Maintenance of Therapeutic Benefit at 10 Months." *Psychosomatic Medicine* 62, no. 5 (September–October 2000): 633–38.

Baker, R. C., and D. S. Kirschenbaum. "Weight Control During the Holidays: Highly Consistent Self-Monitoring as a Potentially Useful Coping Mechanism." *Health Psychology* 17, no. 4 (July 1998): 367–70.

Ballard-Barbash, R., C. M. Friedenreich, K. S. Courneya, S. M. Siddiqi, A. McTiernan, and C. M. Alfano. "Physical Activity, Biomarkers, and Disease Outcomes in Cancer Survivors: A Systematic Review." *Journal of the National Cancer Institute* 104, no. 11 (June 6, 2012): 815–40.

Barone Gibbs B., L. S. Kinzel, K. Pettee Gabriel, Y. F. Chang, and L. H. Kuller. "Short- and Long-Term Eating Habit Modification Predicts Weight Change in Overweight, Postmenopausal Women: Results from the WOMAN Study." *Journal of the Academy of Nutrition and Dietetics* 112, no. 9 (September 2012): 1347–55.

Baumeister, R. F., and J. Tierney. *Willpower: Rediscovering the Greatest Human Strength.* New York: Penguin Press, 2011.

Beers, E. A., J. N. Roemmich, L. H. Epstein, and P. J. Horvath. "Increasing Passive Energy Expenditure during Clerical Work." *European Journal of Applied Physiology* 103, no. 3 (June 2008): 353–60.

Bernstein, M. S., A. Morabia, and D. Sloutskis. "Definition and Prevalence of Sedentarism in an Urban Population." *American Journal of Public Health* 89, no. 6 (June 1999): 862–67.

Bhammar, D. N., S. S. Angadi, and G. A. Gaesser. "Effects of Fractionized and Continuous Exercise on 24-h Ambulatory Blood Pressure." *Medicine and Science in Sports and Exercise* 44, no. 12 (December 2012): 2270–76.

Boutelle, K. N., D. S. Kirschenbaum, R. C. Baker, and M. E. Mitchell. "How Can Obese Weight Controllers Minimize Weight Gain During the High Risk Holiday Season? By Self-Monitoring Very Consistently." *Health Psychology* 18, no. 4 (July 1999): 364–68.

Brown, S. G., and R. E. Rhodes. "Relationships among Dog Ownership and Leisure-Time Walking in Western Canadian Adults." *American Journal of Preventive Medicine* 30, no. 2 (February 2006): 131–36.

Bruusgaard, J. D., I. B. Johansen, I. M. Egner, Z. A. Rana, and K. Gundersen. "Myonuclei Acquired by Overload Exercise Precede Hypertrophy and

Are Not Lost on Detraining." *Proceedings of the National Academy of Sciences* 107, no. 34 (August 24, 2010): 15111–16.

Burgess-Champoux, T. L., N. Larson, D. Neumark-Sztainer, P. J. Hannan, and M. Story. "Are Family Meal Patterns Associated with Overall Diet Quality during the Transition from Early to Middle Adolescence?" *Journal of Nutrition Education and Behavior* 41, no. 2 (March–April 2009): 79–86.

Callahan, P., J. Manier, and D. Alexander. "Where There's Smoke, There Might Be Food Research, Too." *Chicago Tribune*, January 29, 2006, www.chicagotribune.com/business/chi-0601290254jan29,0,1306987.story (accessed 3/20/2013).

Chen, L., L. J. Appel, C. Loria, P. H. Lin, C. M. Champagne, P. J. Elmer, J. D. Ard, D. Mitchell, B. C Batch, L. P. Svetkey, and B. Caballero. "Reduction in Consumption of Sugar-Sweetened Beverages Is Associated with Weight Loss: The PREMIER Trial." *American Journal of Clinical Nutrition* 89, no. 5 (May 2009): 1299–306.

Chen, R. C., M. S. Lee, Y. H. Chang, and M. L. Wahlqvist. "Cooking Frequency May Enhance Survival in Taiwanese Elderly." *Public Health Nutrition* 15, no. 7 (July 2012): 1142–49.

Chiuve, S. E., K. M. Rexrode, D. Spiegelman, G. Logroscino, J. E. Manson, and E. B. Rimm. "Primary Prevention of Stroke by Healthy Lifestyle." *Circulation* 118, no. 9 (August 26, 2008): 947–54.

Chiuve, S. E., L. Sampson, and W. C. Willett. "The Association between a Nutritional Quality Index and Risk of Chronic Disease." *American Journal of Preventive Medicine* 40, no 5 (May 2011): 505–13.

Chuang, S. C., T. Norat, N. Murphy, A. Olsen, A. Tionneland, K. Overvad, M. C. Boutron-Ruault, F. Perquier, L. Dartois, R. Kaaks, B. Teucher, M. M. Bergmann, H. Boeing, A. Trichopoulou, P. Lagiou, D. Trichopoulos, S. Grioni, C. Sacerdote, S. Panico, D. Palli, R. Tumino, P. H. Peeters, B. Bueno-de-Mesquita, M. M. Ros, M. Brustad, L. A. Asli, G. Skeie, J. R., Quirós, C. A., González, M. J. Sánchez, C. Navarro, E. Ardanaz Aicua, M. Dorronsoro, I. Drake, E. Sonestedt, I. Johansson, G. Hallmans, T. Key, F. Crowe, K. T. Khaw, N. Wareham, P. Ferrari, N. Slimani, I. Romieu, V. Gallo, E. Riboli, P. Vineis. "Fiber Intake and Total and Cause-Specific Mortality in the European Prospective Investigation into Cancer and Nutrition Cohort." *American Journal of Clinical Nutrition* 96, no. 1 (July 2012): 164–74.

Church, T. S., D. M. Thomas, C. Tudor-Locke, P. T. Katzmarzyk, C. P. Earnest, R. Q. Rodarte, C. K. Martin, S. N. Blair, and C. Bouchard. "Trends over 5 Decades in U.S. Occupation-Related Physical Activity and Their Associations with Obesity." *PLoS One* 6, no. 5 (2011): e19657.

Coe, D. P., J. M. Pivarnik, C. J. Womack, M. J. Reeves, and R. M. Malina. "Health-Related Fitness and Academic Achievement in Middle School Students." *Journal of Sports Medicine and Physical Fitness* 62, no. 6 (December 2012): 654–60.

Condrasky, M., J. H. Ledikwe, J. E. Flood, and B. J. Rolls. "Chefs' Opinions of Restaurant Portion Sizes." *Obesity* 15, no. 8 (August 2007): 2086–94.

Cooper, S. B., S. Bandelow, and M. E. Nevill. "Breakfast Consumption and Cognitive Function in Adolescent Schoolchildren." *Physiology and Behavior* 103, no. 5 (July 6, 2011): 431–39.

Cox, R. H., J. Guth, L. Siekemeyer, B. Kellems, S. B. Brehm, and C. M. Ohlinger. "Metabolic Cost and Speech Quality while Using an Active Workstation." *Journal of Physical Activity and Health* 8, no. 3 (March 2011): 332–39.

Crowe, F. L., T. J. Key, P. N. Appleby, K. Overvad, E. B. Schmidt, R. Egeberg, A. Tjønneland, R. Kaaks, B. Teucher, H. Boeing, C. Weikert, A. Trichopoulou, V. Ouranos, E. Valanou, G. Masala, S. Sieri, S. Panico, R. Tumino, G. Matullo, H. B. Bueno-de-Mesquita, J. M. Boer, J. W. Beulens, Y. T. van der Schouw, J. R. Quirós, G. Buckland, M. J. Sánchez, M. Dorronsoro, J. M. Huerta, C. Moreno-Iribas, B. Hedblad, J. H. Jansson, P. Wennberg, K. T. Khaw, N. Wareham, P. Ferrari, A. K. Illner, S. C. Chuang, T. Norat, J. Danesh, and E. Riboli. "Dietary Fibre Intake and Ischaemic Heart Disease Mortality: The European Prospective Investigation into Cancer and Nutrition-Heart Study." *European Journal of Clinical Nutrition* 66, no. 8 (August 2012): 950–56.

Crum, A. J., W. R. Corbin, K. D. Brownell, and P. Salovey. "Mind over Milkshakes: Mindsets, Not Just Nutrients, Determine Ghrelin Response." *Health Psychology* 30, no. 4 (July 2011): 424–29.

Csikszentmihalyi, M. *Flow: The Psychology of Optimal Experience.* New York: Harper and Row, 1990.

Daar, A. S., P. A. Singer, D. L. Persad, S. K. Pramming, D. R. Matthews, R. Beaglehole, A. Bernstein, L. K. Borysiewicz, S. Colagiuri, N. Ganguly, R. I. Glass, D. T. Finegood, J. Koplan, E. G. Nabel, G. Sarna, N. Sarrafzadegan, R. Smith, D. Yach, and J. Bell. "Grand Challenges in Chronic Non-Communicable Diseases." *Nature* 450, no. 7169 (November 22, 2007): 494–96.

Davies, N. J., L. Batehup, and R. Thomas. "The Role of Diet and Physical Activity in Breast, Colorectal, and Prostate Cancer Survivorship: A Review of the Literature." *British Journal of Cancer* 105 (2011): S52–S73.

Davis, C. L., N. K. Pollock, J. L. Waller, J. D. Allison, B. A. Dennis, R. Bassali, A. Meléndez, C. A. Boyle, and B. A. Gower. "Exercise Dose and Diabetes Risk in Overweight and Obese Children: A Randomized Controlled Trial." *JAMA* 308, no. 11 (September 19, 2012): 1103–12.

De Castro, J. M., G. A. King, M. Duarte-Gardea, S. Gonzalez-Ayala, and C. H. Kooshian. "Overweight and Obese Humans Overeat Away from Home." *Appetite* 59, no. 2 (October 2012): 204–11.

DeFina, L. F., B. L. Willis, N. B. Radford, A. Gao, D. Leonard, W. L. Haskell, M. F. Weiner, and J. D. Berry. "The Association between Midlife Cardiorespiratory Fitness Levels and Later-Life Dementia: A Cohort Study." *Annals of Internal Medicine* 158, no. 3 (February 5, 2013): 162–68.

Eaton, S. B., L. Cordain, and P. B. Sparling. "Evolution, Body Composition, Insulin Receptor Competition, and Insulin Resistance." *Preventive Medicine* 49, no. 4 (October 2009): 283–85.

Eaton, S. B., S. B. Eaton III, and M. J. Konner. "Paleolithic Nutrition Revisited: A Twelve-Year Retrospective on Its Nature and Implications." *European Journal of Clinical Nutrition* 51, no. 4 (April 1997): 207–16.

Eaton, S. B., S. B. Eaton III, M. J. Konner, and M. Shostak. "An Evolutionary Perspective Enhances Understanding of Human Nutritional Requirements." *Journal of Nutrition* 126, no. 6 (June 1996): 1732–40.

Eaton, S. B., and M. Konner. "Paleolithic Nutrition. A Consideration of Its Nature and Current Implications." *New England Journal of Medicine* 312, no. 5 (January 31, 1985): 283–89.

Ebbeling, C. B., J. F. Swain, H. A. Feldman, W. W. Wong, D. L. Hachey, E. Garcia-Lago, and D. S. Ludwig. "Effects of Dietary Composition on Energy Expenditure during Weight-Loss Maintenance." *JAMA* 307, no. 24 (June 27, 2012): 2627–34.

Ford, E. S., M. M. Bergmann, J. Kröger, A. Schienkiewitz, C. Weikert, and H. Boeing. "Healthy Living Is the Best Revenge: Findings from the European Prospective Investigation into Cancer and Nutrition—Potsdam

Study." *Archives of Internal Medicine* 169, no. 15 (August 10, 2009): 1355–62.

"Four Healthy Lifestyle Factors Help Ward off Chronic Disease: Diet, Exercise, Low Body Mass Index and Not Smoking Can Reduce the Incidence of Heart Disease, Diabetes, Stroke and Cancer." *Duke Medicine Health News* 15, no. 11 (November 2009): 4–5.

"Four Steps to Lower the Toll of Killer Diseases." *Heart Advisor* 7, no. 8 (August 2004): 2.

Framson, C., A. R. Kristal, J. M. Schenk, A. J. Littman, S. Zeliadt, and D. Benitez. "Development and Validation of the Mindful Eating Questionnaire." *Journal of the American Dietetic Association* 109, no. 8 (August 2009): 1439–44.

French, D. P., A. Stevenson, and S. Michie. "An Intervention to Increase Walking Requires Both Motivational and Volitional Components: A Replication and Extension." *Psychology, Health and Medicine* 17, no. 2 (2012): 127–35.

Friedman, E. M., A. S. Karlamangla, D. M. Almeida, and T. E. Seeman. "Social Strain and Cortisol Regulation in Midlife in the U.S." *Social Science and Medicine* 74, no. 4 (February 2012): 607–15.

Furie, G. L., and M. M. Desai. "Active Transportation and Cardiovascular Disease Risk Factors in U.S. Adults." *American Journal of Preventive Medicine* 43, no. 6 (December 2012): 621–28.

Galimanis, A., M. L. Mono, M. Arnold, K. Nedeltchev, and H. P. Mattle. "Lifestyle and Stroke Risk: A Review." *Current Opinion in Neurology* 22, no. 1 (February 2009): 60–68.

Gano, L. B., A. J. Donato, G. L. Pierce, H. M. Pasha, K. A. Magerko, C. Roeca, and D. R. Seals. "Increased Proinflammatory and Oxidant Gene Expression in Circulating Mononuclear Cells in Older Adults: Amelioration by Habitual Exercise." *Physiological Genomics* 43, no. 14 (July 27, 2011): 895–902.

Gaziano, J. M., H. D. Sesso, W. G. Christen, V. Bubes, J. P. Smith, J. MacFadyen, M. Schvartz, J. E. Manson, R. J. Glynn, and J. E. Buring. "Multivitamins in the Prevention of Cancer in Men: The Physicians' Health Study II Randomized Controlled Trial." *JAMA* 308, no. 18 (November 14, 2012): 1871–80.

Glanz, K., J. Hersey, S. Cates, M. Muth, D. Creel, J. Nicholls, V. Fulgoni III, and S. Zaripheh. "Effect of a Nutrient Rich Foods Consumer Education Program: Results from the Nutrition Advice Study." *Journal of the Academy of Nutrition and Dietetics* 112, no. 1 (January 2012): 56–63.

Gopinath, B., E. Rochtchina, V. M. Flood, and P. Mitchell. "Healthy Living and Risk of Major Chronic Diseases in an Older Population." *Archives of Internal Medicine* 170, no. 2 (January 25, 2010): 208–9.

Graham, D. J., and M. N. Laska. "Nutrition Label Use Partially Mediates the Relationship between Attitude toward Healthy Eating and Overall Dietary Quality among College Students." *Journal of the Academy of Nutrition and Dietetics* 112, no. 3 (March 2012): 414–18.

Gregg, E. W., H. Chen, L. E. Wagenknecht, J. M. Clark, L. M. Delahanty, J. Bantle, H. J. Pownall, K. C. Johnson, M. M. Safford, A. E. Kitabchi, F. X. Pi-Sunyer, R. R. Wing, and A. G. Bertoni. "Look AHEAD Research Group. Association of an Intensive Lifestyle Intervention with Remission of Type 2 Diabetes." *JAMA* 308, no. 23 (December 19, 2012): 2489–96.

Groesz, L. M., S. McCoy, J. Carl, L. Saslow, J. Stewart, N. Adler, B. Laraia, and E. Epel. "What Is Eating You? Stress and the Drive to Eat." *Appetite* 58, no. 2 (April 2012): 717–21.

Gupta, B. P., M. H. Murad, M. M. Clifton, L. Prokop, A. Nehra, and S. L. Kopecky. "The Effect of Lifestyle Modification and Cardiovascular Risk Factor Reduction on Erectile Dysfunction: A Systematic Review and Meta-analysis." *Archives of Internal Medicine* 171, no. 20 (November 14, 2011): 1797–803.

Hanlon, B., M. J. Larson, B. W. Bailey, and J. D. Lecheminant. "Neural Response to Pictures of Food after Exercise in Normal-Weight and Obese Women." *Medicine and Science in Sports and Exercise* 44, no. 10 (October 2012): 1864–70.

Heim, S., J. Stang, and M. Ireland. "A Garden Pilot Project Enhances Fruit and Vegetable Consumption among Children." *Journal of the American Dietetic Association* 109, no. 7 (July 2009): 1220–26.

Hermans, R. C., J. K. Larsen, C. P. Herman, and R. C. Engels. "How Much Should I Eat? Situational Norms Affect Young Women's Food Intake during Meal Time." *British Journal of Nutrition* 107, no. 4 (February 2012): 588–94.

Herring, M. P., M. L. Jacob, C. Suveg, R. K. Dishman, and P. J. O'Connor.

"Feasibility of Exercise Training for the Short-Term Treatment of Generalized Anxiety Disorder: A Randomized Controlled Trial." *Psychotherapy and Psychosomatics* 81, no. 1 (2012): 21–28.

Hetherington, M. M., R. Foster, T. Newman, A. S. Anderson, and G. Norton. "Understanding Variety: Tasting Different Foods Delays Satiation." *Physiology and Behavior* 87, no. 2 (February 28, 2006): 263–71.

Hoffman, B. M., M. A. Babyak, W. E. Craighead, A. Sherwood, P. M. Doraiswamy, M. J. Coons, and J. A. Blumenthal. "Exercise and Pharmacotherapy in Patients with Major Depression: One-Year Follow-up of the SMILE Study." *Psychosomatic Medicine* 73, no. 2 (February–March 2011): 127–33.

Institute of Medicine. "Accelerating Progress in Obesity Prevention: Solving the Weight of the Nation." National Academies Report, May 8, 2012, www.iom.edu/Reports/2012/Accelerating-Progress-in-Obesity -Prevention.aspx (accessed 3/20/2013).

Jha, P., C. Ramasundarahettige, V. Landsman, B. Rostron, M. Thun, R. N. Anderson, T. McAfee, and R. Peto. "21st-Century Hazards of Smoking and Benefits of Cessation in the United States." *The New England Journal of Medicine* 368, no. 4 (January 24, 2013): 341–50.

Katz, D. L. "Behavior Modification in Primary Care: The Pressure System Model." *Preventive Medicine* 32, no. 1 (January 2001): 66–72.

———. "Competing Dietary Claims for Weight Loss: Finding the Forest through Truculent Trees." *Annual Review of Public Health* 26 (2005): 61–88.

———. "Life and Death, Knowledge and Power: Why Knowing What Matters Is Not What's the Matter." *Archives of Internal Medicine* 169, no. 15 (August 10, 2009): 1362–63.

———. *Nutrition in Clinical Practice, Second Edition.* Philadelphia: Lippincott Williams and Wilkins, 2008.

———. "Obesity . . . Be Dammed!: What It Will Take to Turn the Tide." *Harvard Health Policy Review* 7 (2006): 135–51.

———. "Pandemic Obesity and the Contagion of Nutritional Nonsense." *Public Health Reviews* 31, no. 1 (2003): 33–44.

———. "Plant Foods in the American Diet? As We Sow . . ." *Medscape Journal of Medicine* 11, no. 1 (2009): 25. Epub January 26, 2009.

———. "School-Based Interventions for Health Promotion and Weight Control: Not Just Waiting on the World to Change." *Annual Review of Public Health* 30 (2009): 253–72.

———. *The Flavor Point Diet: The Delicious, Breakthrough Plan to Turn Off Your Hunger and Lose the Weight for Good.* New York: Rodale Inc., 2005.

———. "2011 Lenna Frances Cooper Memorial Lecture: The Road to Health Is Paved with Good Inventions: Of Science, Sense, and Elephense." *Journal of the Academy of Nutrition and Dietetics* 112, no. 2 (February 2012): 313–21.

Katz, D. L., J. Boukhalil, S. C. Lucan, D. Shah, W. Chan, and M. C. Yeh. "Impediment Profiling for Smoking Cessation. Preliminary Experience." *Behavior Modification* 27, no. 4 (September 2003): 524–37.

Katz, D. L., D. Cushman, J. Reynolds, V. Njike, J. A. Treu, J. Walker, E. Smith, and C. Katz. "Putting Physical Activity Where It Fits in the School Day: Preliminary Results of the ABC (Activity Bursts in the Classroom) for Fitness Program." *Preventing Chronic Disease* 7, no. 4 (July 2010): A82. Epub June 15, 2010.

Katz, D. L., K. Doughty, V. Njike, J. A. Treu, J. Reynolds, J. Walker, E. Smith, and C. Katz. "A Cost Comparison of More and Less Nutritious Food Choices in US Supermarkets." *Public Health Nutrition.* 14, no. 9 (September 2011): 1693–99.

Katz, D. L., and M. H. Gonzalez. *The Way to Eat.* Naperville, IL: Sourcebooks, Inc., 2002.

Katz, D. L., C. S. Katz, J. A. Treu, J. Reynolds, V. Njike, J. Walker, E. Smith, and J. Michael. "Teaching Healthful Food Choices to Elementary School Students and Their Parents: The Nutrition Detectives™ Program." *Journal of School Health* 81, no. 1 (January 2011): 21–28.

Katz, D. L., V. Y. Njike, Z. Faridi, L. Q. Rhee, R. S. Reeves, D. J. Jenkins, and K. T. Ayoob. "The Stratification of Foods on the Basis of Overall Nutritional Quality: The Overall Nutritional Quality Index." *American Journal of Health Promotion* 24, no. 2 (November–December 2009): 133–43.

Katz, D. L., M. O'Connell, V. Y. Njike, M. C. Yeh, H. Nawaz. "Strategies for the Prevention and Control of Obesity in the School Setting: Systematic Review and Meta-analysis." *International Journal of Obesity* 32, no. 12 (December 2008): 1780–89.

Katz, D. L., M. O'Connell, M. C. Yeh, H. Nawaz, V. Njike, L. M. Anderson, S. Cory, and W. Dietz (Task Force on Community Preventive Services). "Public Health Strategies for Preventing and Controlling Overweight and Obesity in School and Worksite Settings: A Report on Recommendations of the Task Force on Community Preventive Services." *Morbidity and Mortality Weekly Report Recommendations and Reports*. 54, no. RR-10 (October 7, 2005): 1–12.

Katz, D. L., K. Shuval, B. P. Comerford, Z. Faridi, and V. Y. Njike. "Impact of an Educational Intervention on Internal Medicine Residents' Physical Activity Counselling: The Pressure System Model." *Journal of Evaluation in Clinical Practice* 14, no. 2 (April 2008): 294–99.

Katzmarzyk, P. T., and I. M. Lee. "Sedentary Behavior and Life Expectancy in the U.S.A.: A Cause-Deleted Life Table Analysis." *British Medical Journal* 2, no. 4 (2012).

Keskitalo, K., H. Tuorila, T. D. Spector, L. F. Cherkas, A. Knaapila, K. Silventoinen, and M. Perola. "Same Genetic Components Underlie Different Measures of Sweet Taste Preference." *American Journal of Clinical Nutrition* 86, no. 6 (December 2007): 1663–69.

Kessler, D. A. *The End of Overeating: Taking Control of the Insatiable American Appetite.* New York: Rodale Books, 2009.

King, D. E., A. G. Mainous III, M. Carnemolla, and C. J. Everett. "Adherence to Healthy Lifestyle Habits in U.S. Adults, 1988–2006." *American Journal of Medicine* 122, no. 6 (June 2009): 528–34.

Knoops, K. T., L. C. de Groot, D. Kromhout, A. E. Perrin, O. Moreiras-Varela, A. Menotti, and W. A. van Staveren. "Mediterranean Diet, Lifestyle Factors, and 10-Year Mortality in Elderly European Men and Women: The HALE Project." *JAMA*. 292, no. 12 (September 22, 2004): 1433–39.

Kong, A., S. A. Beresford, C. M. Alfano, K. E. Foster-Schubert, M. L. Neuhouser, D. B. Johnson, C. Duggan, C. Y. Wang, L. Xiao, R. W. Jeffery, C. E. Bain, and A. McTiernan. "Self-Monitoring and Eating-Related Behaviors Are Associated with 12-Month Weight Loss in Postmenopausal Overweight-to-Obese Women." *Journal of the Academy of Nutrition and Dietetics* 112, no. 9 (September 2012): 1428–35.

Konner, M., and S. B. Eaton. "Paleolithic Nutrition: Twenty-Five Years Later." *Nutrition in Clinical Practice* 25, no. 6 (December 2010): 594–602.

Kovelis, D., J. Zabatiero, K. C. Furlanetto, L. C. Mantoani, M. Proenca, and F. Pitta. "Short-Term Effects of Using Pedometers to Increase Daily Physical Activity in Smokers: A Randomized Trial." *Respiratory Care* 57, no. 7 (July 2012): 1089–97.

Kramer, R. F., A. J. Coutinho, E. Vaeth, K. Christiansen, S. Suratkar, and J. Gittelsohn. "Healthier Home Food Preparation Methods and Youth and Caregiver Psychosocial Factors Are Associated with Lower BMI in African American Youth." *Journal of Nutrition* 142, no. 5 (May 2012): 948–54.

Kuipers, R. S., M. F. Luxwolda, D. A. Dijck-Brouwer, S. B. Eaton, M. A. Crawford, L. Cordain, and F. A. Muskiet. "Estimated Macronutrient and Fatty Acid Intakes from an East African Paleolithic Diet." *British Journal of Nutrition* 104, no. 11 (December 2010): 1666–87.

Kurth, T., S. C. Moore, J. M. Gaziano, C. S. Kase, M. J. Stampfer, K. Berger, and J. E. Buring. "Healthy Lifestyle and the Risk of Stroke in Women." *Archives of Internal Medicine* 166, no. 13 (July 10, 2006): 1403–9.

Kvaavik, E., G. D. Batty, G. Ursin, R. Huxley, and C. R. Gale. "Influence of Individual and Combined Health Behaviors on Total and Cause-Specific Mortality in Men and Women: The United Kingdom Health and Lifestyle Survey." *Archives of Internal Medicine* 170, no. 8 (April 26, 2010): 711–18.

Lapointe, A., V. Provencher, S. J. Weisnagel, C. Bégin, R. Blanchet, A. A. Dufour-Bouchard, C. Trudeau, and S. Lemieux. "Dietary Intervention Promoting High Intakes of Fruits and Vegetables: Short-Term Effects on Eating Behaviors in Overweight-Obese Postmenopausal Women." *Eating Behaviors* 11, no. 4 (December 2010): 305–8.

Larson, N. I., M. C. Nelson, D. Neumark-Sztainer, M. Story, and P. J. Hannan. "Making Time for Meals: Meal Structure and Associations with Dietary Intake in Young Adults." *Journal of the American Dietetic Association* 109, no. 1 (January 2009): 72–79.

Larson, N., D. Neumark-Sztainer, M. N. Laska, and M. Story. "Young Adults and Eating Away from Home: Associations with Dietary Intake Patterns and Weight Status Differ by Choice of Restaurant." *Journal of the American Dietetic Association* 111, no. 11 (November 2011): 1696–703.

Laska, M. N., N. I. Larson, D. Neumark-Sztainer, and M. Story. "Does Involvement in Food Preparation Track from Adolescence to Young

Adulthood and Is It Associated with Better Dietary Quality? Findings from a 10-Year Longitudinal Study." *Public Health Nutrition* 15, no. 7 (July 2012): 1150–58.

Lee, I. M., E. J. Shiroma, F. Lobelo, P. Puska, S. N. Blair, and P. T. Katzmarzyk (Lancet Physical Activity Series Working Group). "Effect of Physical Inactivity on Major Non-communicable Diseases Worldwide: An Analysis of Burden of Disease and Life Expectancy." *Lancet* 380, no. 9838 (July 21, 2012): 219–29.

Lentino, C., A. J. Visek, K. McDonnell, and L. DiPietro. "Dog Walking Is Associated with a Favorable Risk Profile Independent of Moderate to High Volume of Physical Activity." *Journal of Physical Activity and Health* 9, no. 3 (March 2012): 414–20.

Levine, J. A., and J. M. Miller. "The Energy Expenditure of Using a 'Walk-and-Work' Desk for Office Workers with Obesity." *British Journal of Sports Medicine* 41, 9 (September 2007): 558–61.

Levine, J. A., S. J. Schleusner, and M. D. Jensen. "Energy Expenditure of Nonexercise Activity." *American Journal of Clinical Nutrition* 72, no. 6 (December 2000): 1451–54.

Liu, P. J., C. A. Roberto, L. J. Liu, and K. D. Brownell. "A Test of Different Menu Labeling Presentations." *Appetite* 59, no. 3 (December 2012): 770–77.

Loprinzi, P. D., and B. J. Cardinal. "Association between Biologic Outcomes and Objectively Measured Physical Activity Accumulated in >10-Minute Bouts and <10-Minute Bouts." *American Journal of Health Promotion* 27, no. 3 (January–February 2013): 143–51.

Loureiro, M. L., S. T. Yen, and R. M. Nayga Jr. "The Effects of Nutritional Labels on Obesity." *Agricultural Economics* 43, no. 3 (May 2012): 333–42.

McCullough, M. L., A. V. Patel, L. H. Kushi, R. Patel, W. C. Willett, C. Doyle, M. J. Thun, and S. M. Gapstur. "Following Cancer Prevention Guidelines Reduces Risk of Cancer, Cardiovascular Disease, and All-Cause Mortality." *Cancer Epidemiology, Biomarkers and Prevention* 20, no. 6 (June 2011): 1089–97.

McDonald, N. C., A. L. Brown, L. M. Marchetti, and M. S. Pedroso. "U.S. School Travel, 2009: An Assessment of Trends." *American Journal of Preventive Medicine* 41, no. 2 (2011): 146–51.

McGinnis, J. M., and W. H. Foege. "Actual Causes of Death in the United States." *JAMA*. 270, no. 18 (November 10, 1993): 2207–12.

McGonigal, K. *The Willpower Instinct: How Self-Control Works, Why It Matters, and What You Can Do to Get More of It.* New York: Penguin Group, 2012.

Manier, J., P. Callahan, and D. Alexander. "The Oreo, Obesity and Us: A Tribune Special Report in Three Parts." *Chicago Tribune*, August 21–23, 2005, www.chicagotribune.com/news/watchdog/chi-oreos-specialpackage ,0,6758724.special (accessed 3/20/2013).

Meng, L., G. Maskarinec, J. Lee, and L. N. Kolonel. "Lifestyle Factors and Chronic Diseases: Application of a Composite Risk Index." *Preventive Medicine* 29, no. 4 (October 1999): 296–304.

Meyer, P., B. Kayser, M. P. Kossovsky, P. Sigaud, D. Carballo, P. F. Keller, X. E. Martin, N. Farpour-Lambert, C. Pichard, and F. Mach. "Stairs Instead of Elevators at Workplace: Cardioprotective Effects of a Pragmatic Intervention." *European Journal of Cardiovascular Prevention and Rehabilitation* 17, no. 5 (October 2010): 569–75.

Mokdad, A. H., J. S. Marks et al. "Actual Causes of Death in the United States, 2000." *JAMA*. 291, no. 10 (March 10, 2004): 1238–45. Review. Erratum in *JAMA* 293, no. 3 (January 19, 2005): 293–94.

Muchiteni, T., and W. B. Borden. "Improving Risk Factor Modification: A Global Approach." *Current Cardiology Reports*. 11, no. 6 (November 2009): 476–83.

Murawski, M. E., V. A. Milsom, K. M. Ross, K. A. Rickel, N. DeBraganza, L. M. Gibbons, and M. G. Perri. "Problem Solving, Treatment Adherence, and Weight-Loss Outcome among Women Participating in Lifestyle Treatment for Obesity." *Eating Behaviors* 10, no. 3 (August 2009): 146–51.

Myers, K. P., and A. Sclafani. "Development of Learned Flavor Preferences." *Developmental Psychobiology* 48, no. 5 (July 2006): 380–88.

National Diabetes Information Clearinghouse: Diabetes Prevention Program (DPP). http://diabetes.niddk.nih.gov/dm/pubs/preventionprogram/ (accessed 3/20/2013).

Nicklett, E. J., R. D. Semba, Q. L. Xue, J. Tian, K. Sun, A. R. Cappola, E. M. Simonsick, L. Ferrucci, and L. P. Fried. "Fruit and Vegetable Intake, Physical Activity, and Mortality in Older Community-Dwelling

Women." *Journal of the American Geriatrics Society* 60, no. 5 (May 2012): 862–68.

O'Connell, M., B. P. Comerford, H. K. Wall, V. Yanchou-Njike, Z. Faridi, and D. L. Katz. "Impediment Profiling for Smoking Cessation: Application in the Worksite." *American Journal of Health Promotion* 21, 2 (November–December 2006): 97–100.

O'Connell, M., S. C. Lucan, M. C. Yeh, E. Rodriguez, D. Shah, W. Chan, and D. L. Katz. "Impediment Profiling for Smoking Cessation: Results of a Pilot Study." *American Journal of Health Promotion* 17, no. 5 (May–June 2003): 300–303.

O'Keefe, J. H., R. Vogel, C. J. Lavie, and L. Cordain. "Achieving Hunter-Gatherer Fitness in the 21st Century: Back to the Future." *American Journal of Medicine* 123, no. 12 (December 2010): 1082–86.

———. "Organic Fitness: Physical Activity Consistent with Our Hunter-Gatherer Heritage." *Physician and Sportsmedicine.* 38, no. 4 (December 2010): 11–18.

Ogden, L. G., N. Stroebele, H. R. Wyatt, V. A. Catenacci, J. C. Peters, J. Stuht, R. R. Wing, and J. O. Hill. "Cluster Analysis of the National Weight Control Registry to Identify Distinct Subgroups Maintaining Successful Weight Loss." *Obesity* 20, no. 10 (October 2012): 2039–47.

Ornish, D., S. E. Brown, L. W. Scherwitz, J. H. Billings, W. T. Armstrong, T. A. Ports, S. M. McLanahan, R. L. Kirkeeide, R. J. Brand, and K. L. Gould. "Can Lifestyle Changes Reverse Coronary Heart Disease? The Lifestyle Heart Trial." *The Lancet* 336, no. 8708 (July 21, 1990): 129–33.

Ornish, D, J. Lin, J. Daubenmier, G. Weidner, E. Epel, C. Kemp, M. J. Magbanua, R. Marlin, L. Yglecias, P. R. Carroll, and E. H. Blackburn. "Increased Telomerase Activity and Comprehensive Lifestyle Changes: A Pilot Study." *The Lancet Oncology* 9, no. 11 (November 2008): 1048–57.

Ornish, D, M. J. Magbanua, G. Weidner, V. Weinberg, C. Kemp, C. Green, M. D. Mattie, R. Marlin, J. Simko, K. Shinohara, C. M. Haqq, and P. R. Carroll. "Changes in Prostate Gene Expression in Men Undergoing an Intensive Nutrition and Lifestyle Intervention." *Proceedings of the National Academy of Sciences U.S.A.* 105, no. 24 (June 17, 2008): 8369–74.

Ornish, D, L. W. Scherwitz, J. H. Billings, S. E. Brown, K. L. Gould, T. A. Merritt, S. Sparler, W. T. Armstrong, T. A. Ports, R. L. Kirkeeide, C. Hogeboom, R. J. Brand, et al. "Intensive Lifestyle Changes for Reversal of Coronary Heart Disease." *JAMA* 280, no. 23 (December 16, 1998): 2001–7.

Orrell-Valente, J. K., L. G. Hill, W. A. Brechwald, K. A. Dodge, G. S. Pettit, and J. E. Bates. "'Just Three More Bites': An Observational Analysis of Parents' Socialization of Children's Eating at Mealtime." *Appetite* 48, no. 1 (January 2007): 37–45.

Park, M. "Twinkie Diet Helps Nutrition Professor Lose 27 Pounds." *CNN*, November 8, 2010, www.cnn.com/2010/HEALTH/11/08/twinkie.diet .professor/index.html (accessed 3/20/2013).

Parschau, L., L. Fleig, M. Koring, D. Lange, N. Knoll, R. Schwarzer, and S. Lippke. "Positive Experience, Self-Efficacy, and Action Control Predict Physical Activity Changes: A Moderated Mediation Analysis." *British Journal of Health Psychology*, 18, no. 2, May 2013: 395-406.

Pecoraro, N., F. Reyes, F. Gomez, A. Bhargava, and M. F. Dallman. "Chronic Stress Promotes Palatable Feeding, Which Reduces Signs of Stress: Feedforward and Feedback Effects of Chronic Stress." *Endocrinology* 145, no. 8 (August 2004): 3754–62.

Pollan, M. *In Defense of Food: An Eater's Manifesto.* New York: Penguin Press, 2008.

Prochaska, J. O., J. C. Norcross, and C. C. DiClemente. *Changing for Good: A Revolutionary Six-Stage Program for Overcoming Bad Habits and Moving Your Life Positively Forward.* New York: William Morrow and Company, 1994.

Ramsden, C. E., K. R. Faurot, P. Carrera-Bastos, L. Cordain, M. De Lorgeril, and L. S. Sperling. "Dietary Fat Quality and Coronary Heart Disease Prevention: A Unified Theory Based on Evolutionary, Historical, Global, and Modern Perspectives." *Current Treatment Options in Cardiovascular Medicine* 11, no. 4 (August 2009): 289–301.

Ramsey, F., A. Ussery-Hall, D. Garcia, G. McDonald, A. Easton, M. Kambon, L. Balluz, W. Garvin, and J. Vigeant. "Prevalence of Selected Risk Behaviors and Chronic Diseases—Behavioral Risk Factor Surveillance System (BRFSS), 39 Steps Communities, United States, 2005." *Morbidity and Mortality Weekly Report Surveillance Summary* 57, no. 11 (October 31, 2008): 1–20.

Ratey, J. J., and E. Hagerman. *Spark: The Revolutionary New Science of Exercise and the Brain.* New York: Little, Brown and Company, 2008.

Razquin, C., J. A. Martinez, M. A. Martinez-Gonzalez, J. Fernández-Creheut, J. M. Santos, and A. Marti. "A Mediterranean Diet Rich in Virgin Olive Oil May Reverse the Effects of the -174G/C IL6 Gene Variant on 3-Year Body Weight Change." *Molecular Nutrition and Food Research* 54, suppl. 1 (May 2010): S75–82.

Razquin, C., J. A. Martinez, M. A. Martinez-Gonzalez, M. T. Mitjavila, R. Estruch, and A. Marti. "A 3 Years Follow-Up of a Mediterranean Diet Rich in Virgin Olive Oil Is Associated with High Plasma Antioxidant Capacity and Reduced Body Weight Gain." *European Journal of Clinical Nutrition* 63, no. 12 (December 2009): 1387–93.

Reynolds, G. *The First 20 Minutes: Surprising Science Reveals How We Can Exercise Better, Train Smarter, Live Longer.* New York: Hudson Street Press, 2012.

Robert Wood Johnson Foundation. "Declining Childhood Obesity Rates—Where Are We Seeing the Most Progress?" *Health Policy Snapshot*, September 2012, www.rwjf.org/content/dam/farm/reports/issue_briefs/2012/rwjf401163. (accessed 3/20/2013).

Roberts, V., R. Maddison, C. Simpson, C. Bullen, and H. Prapavessis. "The Acute Effects of Exercise on Cigarette Cravings, Withdrawal Symptoms, Affect, and Smoking Behaviour: Systematic Review Update and Meta-analysis." *Psychopharmacology* 222 (2012): 1–15.

Robinson, E., J. Blissett, and S. Higgs. "Recall of Vegetable Eating Affects Future Predicted Enjoyment and Choice of Vegetables in British University Undergraduate Students." *Journal of the American Dietetic Association* 111, no. 10 (October 2011): 1543–48.

Rolls, B. J., L. S. Roe, and J. S. Meengs. "Large Portion Sizes Lead to a Sustained Increase in Energy Intake over 2 Days." *Journal of the American Dietetic Association* 106, no. 4 (April 2006): 543–49.

Ruby, M. B., E. W. Dunn, A. Perrino, R. Gillis, and S. Viel. "The Invisible Benefits of Exercise." *Health Psychology* 30, no. 1 (January 2011): 67–74.

Salomon, J. A., H. Wang, M. K. Freeman, T. Vos., A. D. Flaxman, A. D. Lopez, and C. J. Murray. "Healthy Life Expectancy for 187 Countries, 1990–2010: A Systematic Analysis for the Global Burden Disease Study 2010." *The Lancet* 380, no. 9859 (December 15, 2012): 2144–62. Erratum in *The Lancet* 380, no. 9867 (February 23, 2012): 628.

Schwartz, M. B., L. R. Vartanian, C. M. Wharton, and K. D. Brownell. "Examining the Nutritional Quality of Breakfast Cereals Marketed to Children." *Journal of the American Dietetic Association* 108, no. 4 (April 2008): 702–5.

"Shape of the Nation Report 2012." National Association for Sport and Physical Education and the American Heart Association.

Smith, K. J., L. Blizzard, S. A. McNaughton, S. L. Gall, T. Dwyer, and A. J. Venn. "Takeaway Food Consumption and Cardio-Metabolic Risk Factors in Young Adults." *European Journal of Clinical Nutrition.* 66, no. 5 (May 2012): 577–84.

Snyder, A., B. Colvin, and J. K. Gammack. "Pedometer Use Increases Daily Steps and Functional Status in Older Adults." *Journal of the American Medical Directors Association.* 12, no. 8 (October 2011): 590–94.

Spencer, E. A., K. L. Pirie, R. J. Stevens, V. Beral, A. Brown, B. Liu, J. Green, and G. K. Reeves. "Diabetes and Modifiable Risk Factors for Cardiovascular Disease: The Prospective Million Women Study." *European Journal of Epidemiology* 23, no. 12 (2008): 793–99.

Steeves, J. A., D. L. Thompson, and D. R. Bassett Jr. "Energy Cost of Stepping in Place while Watching Television Commercials." *Medicine and Science in Sports and Exercise.* 44, no. 2 (February 2012): 330–35.

Stein, L. J., H. Nagai, M. Nakagawa, and G. K. Beauchamp. "Effects of Repeated Exposure and Health-Related Information on Hedonic Evaluation and Acceptance of a Bitter Beverage." *Appetite.* 40, no. 2 (April 2003): 119–29.

Steptoe, A., and J. Wardle. "What the Experts Think: A European Survey of Expert Opinion about the Influence of Lifestyle on Health." *European Journal of Epidemiology* 10, no. 2 (April 1994): 195–203.

Stroebele, N., and J. M. De Castro. "Effect of Ambience on Food Intake and Food Choice." *Nutrition* 20, no. 9 (September 2004): 821–38.

———. "Listening to Music While Eating Is Related to Increases in People's Food Intake and Meal Duration." *Appetite* 47, no. 3 (November 2006): 285–89.

Sun, X. D., X. E. Liu, and D. S. Huang. "Curcumin Induces Apoptosis of Triple-Negative Breast Cancer Cells by Inhibition of EGFR Expression." *Molecular Medicine Reports* 6, no. 6 (December 2012): 1267–70.

Tanaka, S., S. Yamamoto, M. Inoue, M. Iwasaki, S. Sasazuki, H. Iso, and S. Tsugane. "Projecting the Probability of Survival Free from Cancer and

Cardiovascular Incidence through Lifestyle Modification in Japan." *Preventive Medicine* 48, no. 2 (February 2009): 128–33.

Taylor, A. H., and A. J. Oliver. "Acute Effects of Brisk Walking on Urges to Eat Chocolate, Affect, and Responses to a Stressor and Chocolate Cue: An Experimental Study." *Appetite* 52, no. 1 (February 2009): 155–60.

Turner, S. A., A. Luszczynska, L. Warner, and R. Schwarzer. "Emotional and Uncontrolled Eating Styles and Chocolate Chip Cookie Consumption: A Controlled Trial of the Effects of Positive Mood Enhancement." *Appetite* 54, no. 1 (February 2010): 143–49.

Van der Ploeg, H. P., T. Chey, R. J. Korda, E. Banks, and A. Bauman. "Sitting Time and All-Cause Mortality Risk in 222,497 Australian Adults." *Archives of Internal Medicine* 172, no. 6 (March 26, 2012): 494–500.

Van Dijk, S. J., E. J. Feskens, M. B. Bos, D. W. Hoelen, R. Heijligenberg, M. G. Bromhaar, L. D. de Groot, J. H. de Vries, M. Müller, and L. A. Afman. "A Saturated Fatty Acid-Rich Diet Induces an Obesity-Linked Proinflammatory Gene Expression Profile in Adipose Tissue of Subjects at Risk of Metabolic Syndrome." *American Journal of Clinical Nutrition* 90, no. 6 (December 2009): 1656–64.

Van Kleef, E., M. Shimizu, and B. Wansink. "Food Compensation: Do Exercise Ads Change Food Intake?" *International Journal of Behavioral Nutrition and Physical Activity* 8 (January 28, 2011): 6.

Vartanian, L. R., C. P. Herman, and B. Wansink. "Are We Aware of the External Factors That Influence Our Food Intake?" *Health Psychology* 27, no. 5 (2008): 533–38.

Wallace, J. P., J. S. Raglin, and C. A. Jastremski. "Twelve Month Adherence of Adults Who Joined a Fitness Program with a Spouse vs. without a Spouse." *Journal of Sports Medicine and Physical Fitness* 35, no. 3 (September 1995): 206–13.

Wannamethee, S. G., A. G. Shaper, M. Walker, and S. Ebrahim. "Lifestyle and 15-Year Survival Free of Heart Attack, Stroke, and Diabetes in Middle-Aged British Men." *Archives of Internal Medicine* 158, no. 22 (December 7–21, 1998): 2433–40.

Wansink, B. *Mindless Eating: Why We Eat More Than We Think*. New York: Bantam Dell, 2006.

Warziski, M. T., S. M. Sereika, M. A. Styn, E. Music, and L. E. Burke. "Changes in Self-Efficacy and Dietary Adherence: The Impact on

Weight Loss in the PREFER Study." *Journal of Behavioral Medicine* 31, no. 1 (February 2008): 81–92.

Weisburger, J. H. "Lifestyle, Health and Disease Prevention: The Underlying Mechanisms." *European Journal of Cancer Prevention* 11, suppl. 2 (August 2002): S1–7.

Woo, J. "Relationships among Diet, Physical Activity and Other Lifestyle Factors and Debilitating Diseases in the Elderly." *European Journal of Clinical Nutrition* 54, suppl. 3 (June 2000): S143–47.

Wyse, R., E. Campbell, N. Nathan, and L. Wolfenden. "Associations between Characteristics of the Home Food Environment and Fruit and Vegetable Intake in Preschool Children: A Cross-Sectional Study." *BMC Public Health* 11 (December 16, 2011): 938.

Yeh, M. C., S. B. Ickes, L. M . Lowenstein, K. Shuval, A. S. Ammerman, R. Farris, and D. L. Katz. "Understanding Barriers and Facilitators of Fruit and Vegetable Consumption among a Diverse Multi-ethnic Population in the U.S.A." *Health Promotion International* 23, no. 1 (March 2008): 42–51.

Yeh, M. C., E. Rodriguez, H. Nawaz, M. Gonzalez, D. Nakamoto, and D. L. Katz. "Technical Skills for Weight Loss: 2-Year Follow-Up Results of a Randomized Trial." *International Journal of Obesity and Related Metabolic Disorders* 27, no. 12 (December 2003): 1500–1506.

Yi W., and H. Y. Wetzstein. "Anti-Tumorigenic Activity of Five Culinary and Medicinal Herbs Grown under Greenhouse Conditions and Their Combination Effects." *Journal of the Science of Food and Agriculture* 91, no. 10 (August 15, 2011): 1849–54.

Zhang, Y., and R. Cooke. "Using a Combined Motivational and Volitional Intervention to Promote Exercise and Healthy Dietary Behaviour among Undergraduates." *Diabetes Research and Clinical Practice.* 95, no. 2 (February 2012): 215–23.

Index